D0839086

Other Books by
John Neustadt, ND and Steve Pieczenik, MD, PhD

A Revolution in Health through Nutritional Biochemistry (iUniverse 2007)

A Revolution in Health Part 2: How to Take Charge of Your Health (iUniverse 2009)

Foundations and Applications of Medical Biochemistry in Clinical Practice

By John Neustadt, ND
Steve Pieczenik, MD, PhD

iUniverse, Inc.
New York   Bloomington

Foundations and Applications of Medical Biochemistry in Clinical Practice

iUniverse books may be ordered through booksellers or by contacting:

iUniverse
1663 Liberty Drive
Bloomington, IN 47403
www.iuniverse.com
1-800-Authors (1-800-288-4677)

ISBN: 978-1-4401-2535-5 (pbk)
ISBN: 978-1-4401-2534-8 (ebk)

Printed in the United States of America

iUniverse rev. date: 6/10/09

Dedication

Dr. Pieczenik would like to dedicate this book to his father, Dr. Saul Pieczenik, and his mother, Teodora Janowska Pieczenik, both of whom died an early death. They fled the Holocaust in Europe in order to bring their two sons to the safety of America. And to my wonderful wife, Roberta (Birdie) Pieczenik, PhD, who has been the perfect life companion for me and who has supported and understood my need to continually search out new paradigms in the different careers I've had. To my adventuresome daughter, Sharon Pieczenik, MFA, whose ability to endure the cold of the Arctic and the heat of Madagascar in her quest to make this world a better world through documentary film making is inspirational. To the new doctor in the family, Stephanie Pieczenik, MD, who made history by writing the first textbook by a medical student for *Gray's Anatomy*, and who introduced me to the field of integrative medicine. And to my partner and physician with whom I wrote this book, John Neustadt, ND, who graciously invited me and taught me about a world in medicine far beyond my imagination, and who had the patience to tutor me in the basic alphabet of his biochemical language.

Dr. Neustadt would like to dedicate this book to his wife, Romi, who has endured countless hours away from her husband in his pursuit to bring this revolutionary approach in medicine to a broader audience. She has always had faith in who I am and what I do and has always encouraged me to strive for my dreams. To Nate, the most wonderful boy in the world. In your eyes shine hope, happiness, immeasurable curiosity, and a slight mischievous quality that I adore. And to my newborn daughter, Bebe, who I hope grows up to be strong, self-assured, and to follow her own dreams. May both of my children inherit a world where healthcare is truly based on the Laws of Nature. And of course, to my partner, Dr. Steve Pieczenik, who mentored me in medicine and business and has helped me develop in myself the clinical and interpersonal skills that I could never have even thought were possible.

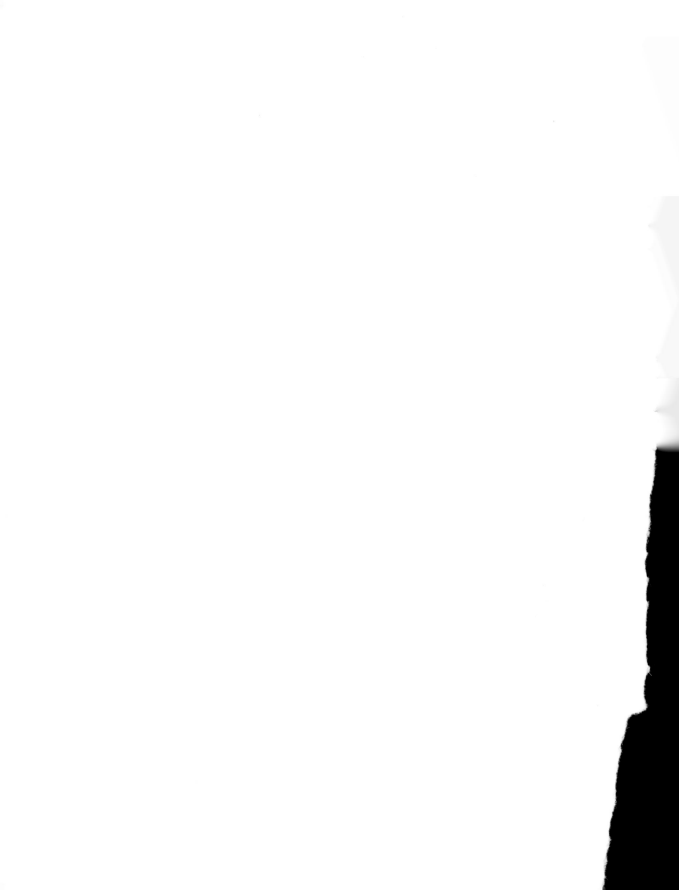

Contents

Foreword

The diagnostic and treatment approaches described in this book are used every day by Dr. Neustadt in his clinic, Montana Integrative Medicine. Dr. Pieczenik does not diagnose or treat patients. His role has been to help define this novel paradigm shift in medicine away from symptoms to underlying biochemical causality, and to ensure that it is developed and widely disseminated. Treatment plans based on Functional Biochemical Testing are meant to provide short-term nutritional support with dietary supplements to replenish nutrients that patients are deficient in while working with them to optimize their diet and lifestyle for long-term health. The foundation of long-term health is not pills and powders, but diet and lifestyle. The dietary supplements are there to help people feel better quickly by "jump starting" their biochemistry and giving the body the nutrients it needs to function.

During the three months on the program, the goal is to improve patients' diet and lifestyle so that as the number of dietary supplements are reduced, diet and lifestyle can take over to maintain and continue to improve health in the long term. This approach also teaches patients how they can better take care of themselves so that they hopefully will not only be cured, but will no longer be dependent on doctors and will prevent future illness.

Frequently patients will ask if they must retake an entire test panel that's ordered, such as the MetaCT 400, which reports more than 450 analytes. The answer is that in the vast majority of cases retesting all the analytes is not necessary. Most variables tested, such as serum amino acids and urinary organic acids correlate with symptoms, such as fatigue, irritability, depression and insomnia. As patients follow their individualized, three-month programs, the crucial issue clinically is not whether an analyte changes during that time, which it does, but whether someone feels better. The bottom line is clinical improvement, not changes in a lab value. Therefore, in most cases retesting is not necessary. However, retesting is necessary to track changes in analytes that do not correspond to symptomatic improvement, but are risk factors for diseases. This is the case for analytes such as elevated lipids, fibrinogen and C-reactive protein (CRP). These are risk factors for cardiovascular disease, and decreasing them when elevated is important for preventing heart disease and strokes. However, changes in lab results over time do not result in changes in how the patient feels. Therefore, retesting these are important.

NBI Functional Biochemical Testing utilizes sophisticated laboratory techniques to identify the underlying biochemical causes of disease. Many times these causes have to do with "subclinical" nutritional deficiencies, which manifest as symptoms but are not recognized by the conventional medical community as playing any role in health and disease progression. The authors, as have others, have come to a different conclusion (Figure i.i).

Figure i.i. Stages of Development of Nutrient-Insufficiency Diseases

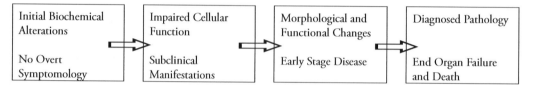

Through a careful medical history and physical examination, and by correcting the underlying biochemical determinants of symptoms as identified through testing, clinicians can promote patients' health and literally cure them. Because this approach identifies the underlying causes of disease that can then be corrected using a Targeted Nutritional Program™ (TNP), it provides hope to patients and real clinical improvements.

How to Use This Book

The following cases are examples of people who have been helped by Dr. Neustadt and his approach of helping people by identifying and treating the underlying causes of illnesses. Since biochemistry is a web of interactions, conditions will have many different symptoms, such as someone complaining of arthritis, fatigue, and depression. In writing up these cases, it was sometimes difficult to decide under which category to put a case. Every effort was made to categorize cases based on the main presenting symptom.

The people suffering from these conditions and symptoms were evaluated by Dr. Neustadt in his clinic, Montana Integrative Medicine. Many of these people already had medical diagnoses, such as depression or mature onset asthma. However, those diagnoses, like most medical diagnoses, do not provide any information about the underlying biochemical causes of the symptoms. Functional Biochemical Testing generates a large amount of data that allows skilled interpreters to provide functional diagnoses. This approach to medicine is aptly called *functional medicine* because it provides a description of the underlying causes of symptoms and diseases and leads to a proactive treatment that treats the underlying cause. With this information, customized plans are created to help restore biochemical balance, alleviate symptoms, and correct the underlying causes of disease.

The authors recommend that readers extensively utilize the appendices and index at the end of the book to fully comprehend topics and diseases they wish to learn about. Dr. Neustadt includes every nutrient in every dietary supplement in a patient's treatment plan, which can be several pages long. He does this so that he knows exactly how much of a given nutrient (e.g., vitamin B6, isoleucine, magnesium) a patient is consuming to ensure that therapeutic and safe doses are obtained. Treatment plans are included in the book so that readers can learn how to apply this approach in clinical practice. However, since listing out every nutrient in every dietary supplement for every treatment plan would be redundant and tedious to read, a full list of nutraceuticals and their ingredients are included in the Appendix B.

Since many different symptoms are associated with different causes, the symptoms will appear in many different cases and section in the book. An example of this is depression, which is a common complaint in many different diseases, such as fatigue, migraine headaches, fibromyalgia, arthritis, seizure disorder, irritable bowel syndrome (IBS), Lyme disease, migraine headaches, and multiple sclerosis.

The conditions in this book were arranged based on the primary complaint of the patient; however, ancillary problems were also charted and treated, so that if a physician is treating a person with IBS and cancer, depression will inevitably come up. Some readers may find it helpful to take a nonlinear approach to studying this book by using the index and studying cases that present with symptoms or diagnoses of interest.

Chapter One

The Neustadt-Pieczenik Paradigm Shift in Medicine

The Neustadt-Pieczenik Paradigm Shift in medicine represents the fusion and clinical applications of biochemistry, thermodynamics, physiology, enzymology, nutritional medicine, and laboratory testing to identify and correct the underlying causes of many diseases that are considered genetic in nature (e.g., Phenylketonuria) as well as those that are not considered genetic (e.g., mature onset asthma, depression, fatigue). In doing so, this paradigm shift presents a heuristic model with intellectual precursors dating as far back as 1902. Since then it has been proven to be effective in numerous clinical trials and case reports. Drs. Neustadt and Pieczenik present for the first time this paradigm shift as a coherent set of constructs for approaching patient diagnosis and treatment through functional biochemical medicine.

History of Medical Biochemistry

Biochemistry is a complex web of interactions involving an interplay among genetics, diet, and lifestyle. One of the earliest works to discuss biochemical individuality was written in 1902. In that year, Archibald E. Garrod, MD, a clinician in London, England, published a paper in the journal *Lancet* detailing observations on patients with alkaptonuria, an autosomal recessive metabolic disorder that results in a decreased ability to metabolize the amino acids phenylalanine and tyrosine. Phenylalanine, an essential amino acid, is metabolized in vivo to tyrosine, which continues down its pathway to eventually become thyroid hormone, melanin, dopamine, and epinephrine. Alkatptonuria results in a defect in the enzyme homogentistic acid oxidase (HGAO), which catalyzes a single step in the metabolism of phenylalanine and tyrosine—the transformation of homogentisic acid (HA) to maleylacetoacetic acid (Figure 1.1). HA is cleared by the kidneys and, upon contact with the air, causes urine to turn black. Oxidation of HA also causes an accumulation of dark pigment in cartilage and skin, called ochronosis, and leads to arthritis in adulthood, particularly in the spine and large joints.

Figure 1.1. Pathway involved in alkaptonuria

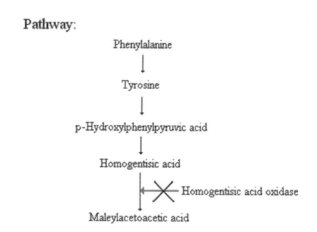

Dr. Garrod reported, "There are good reasons for thinking that alkaptonuria is not the manifestation of a disease but is rather the nature of an alternative course of metabolism…. If it be a correct inference from the available facts that the individuals of a species do not conform to an absolutely rigid standard of metabolism but differ slightly in their chemistry as they do in their structure, it is no more surprising that they should occasionally exhibit conspicuous deviations from the specific type of metabolism than that we should meet with such wide departures from the structural uniformity of the species as the presence of supernumerary digits or transposition of the viscera."[1] This astute observer was able to extrapolate subtle changes in biochemical function to anatomical variations.

It was not until 1956 that Roger Williams, PhD, a pioneer in nutrition often credited with popularizing the term "biochemical individuality," wrote the book *Biochemical Individuality: The Basis for the Genetotrophic Concept.*[2] Williams believed that people have different requirements for nutrients, and some may need much greater quantities of nutrients than others in order for their unique biochemistry to function properly. He wrote, "Individuality in nutritional needs is the basis for the genetotrophic approach and for the belief that nutrition applied with due concern for individual genetic variations, which may be large, offers the solution to many baffling health problems."

Dr. Williams based his assertions on anatomical and physiological variations among individuals, and only in the latter years of the last century would the biochemical bases for these assertions be explained by researchers such as Bruce Ames, PhD, a UC Berkeley biochemist. Dr. Ames applied the concept of Dr. Williams' work to studying gene-nutrient interactions. Dr. Ames' research showed that variations among genes producing the same enzyme for a biochemical reaction commonly decrease the enzyme's binding affinity (its ability to use its cofactors).[3-6]

This binding affinity is described by the Michaelis-Menten equation. This equation was created in 1913 by Leonor Michaelis, MD, a German biochemist and physician, and Maud Menten, MD, PhD, a Canadian who worked with Dr. Michaelis in Germany because women were not allowed to do research in Canada at the time. The Michaelis-Menten equation describes the ability of an enzymatic reaction to create products from reactants. To determine the maximum rate of an enzyme mediated reaction, a series of experiments is carried out where the substrate concentration ($[S]$) is increased until a constant initial rate of product formation is achieved. This is the *maximum velocity* (V_{max}) of the enzyme under the conditions of the experiment. In this state, enzyme active sites are saturated with substrate. The reaction rate V is the number of reactions per second catalyzed per mole of the enzyme. The reaction rate increases with increasing substrate concentration $[S]$, asymptotically approaching the maximum rate V_{max}. There is therefore no clearly-defined substrate concentration at which the enzyme can be said to be saturated with substrate. A more appropriate measure to characterize an enzyme is the substrate concentration at which the reaction rate reaches half of its maximum value ($V_{max}/2$). This concentration can be shown to be equal to the Michaelis constant (K_M).

For enzymatic reactions that exhibit simple Michaelis-Menten kinetics and in which product formation is the rate-limiting step (i.e., when $k_2 << k_{-1}$) $K_m \approx k_{-1}/k_1 = K_d$, where K_d is the dissociation constant (affinity for substrate) of the enzyme-substrate (ES) complex. However, often $k_2 >> k_{-1}$, or k_2 and k_{-1} are comparable, in which case nothing can be said about the enzyme affinity from the Michaelis constant alone.

The Michaelis constant can be defined as:

Figure 1.3. Michaelis constant equation

$$K_m = \frac{k_{-1} + k_2}{k_1}$$

The Michaelis-Menten equation has been the foundation for the study of enzyme kinetics in free-flowing systems and is based on mass-action laws and the assumption of free diffusion. However, the cellular and subcellular environment in human physiology is not a free-flowing system. There are complex transport mechanisms and equations that delineate the biochemical interactions. The Michaelis-Menten equation was the foundation for the study of these biological systems, which has been called *fractal enzymology.*[7]

Despite the limitations of the classic Michaelis-Menten equation, Dr. Ames has successfully applied it to human biological systems and single-nucleotide polymorphisms (SNPs). Genes code for proteins. One class of proteins is enzymes, which catalyze biochemical reactions. This means that they increase the rate at which a reaction occurs. Enzymes are known to catalyze about four thousand biochemical reactions. Most enzymes in biochemical reactions require cofactors, which are inorganic (e.g., metal ions and iron-sulfur clusters) or organic compounds (e.g., flavin and heme).

Enzyme kinetics is the field of study that underlies biochemical function. It describes the rate at which an enzyme is able to convert reactants to products in an *in vivo* environment. A simple enzyme kinetics model that underlies the assumptions in functional biochemical testing is illustrated in the following equation (Figure 1.4).

Figure 1.4. Enzyme kinetics

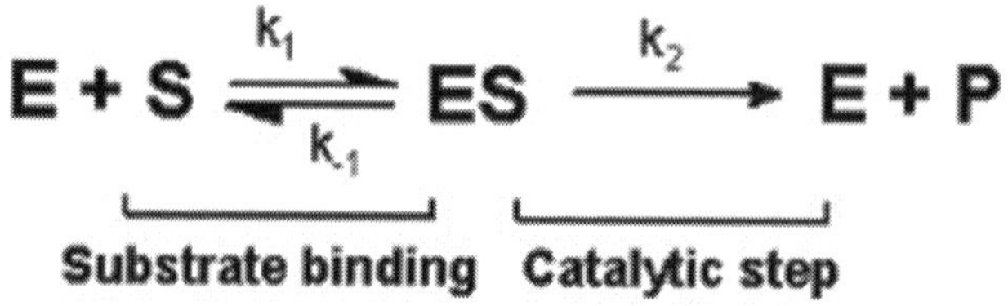

$$E + S \underset{k_{-1}}{\overset{k_1}{\rightleftharpoons}} ES \xrightarrow{k_2} E + P$$

Substrate binding   Catalytic step

In Figure 1.4, E is the enzyme, S is the substrate, ES is the enzyme-substrate complex, P is the product, and k_1, k_2, and k_3 are the constants for individual reactions.

Figure 1.5. Activation energy decreased with enzymes to produce more products over a given time.

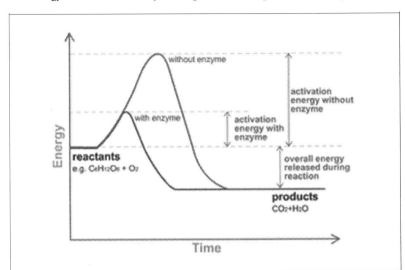

These constants (k_1, k_2, and k_3) reflect the ability of the enzymes to catalyze the reactions. Like all catalysts, enzymes work by lowering the activation energy for a reaction, thus dramatically increasing the rate of the reaction (Figure 1.5). Most enzyme reaction rates are millions of times faster than those of comparable un-catalyzed reactions. As with all catalysts, enzymes are not consumed by the reactions they catalyze, nor do they alter the equilibrium of these reactions. However, enzymes do differ from most other catalysts by being much more specific.

Genetic polymorphisms, medications, hormones (e.g., cholesterol, estrogen), and environmental toxins can alter the reaction constants (k_1, k_2, and k_3). This causes an accumulation of substrates and a decrease in products. Dr. Ames extrapolated from his research to conclude that at least one third of SNPs decrease the ability of a cofactor to bind to and activate its enzyme. This decreases the K(m) and the ability of the enzyme to facilitate a biochemical reaction. The result is an accumulation of reactants and decreased quantities of products.[3-6] This situation can be corrected by providing higher amounts of the cofactors, which effectively pushes the reaction in the direction of products.[3-6]

Phenylketonuria (PKU) provides an excellent illustration of the concept behind functional biochemical testing and why simply testing for a gene is insufficient. PKU is an autosomal recessive genetic disorder that has historically been viewed as irreversible. PKU results from phenylalanine hydroxylase (PAH) deficiency.[8] PAH catalyzes the reaction of phenylalanine

(Phe), the reactant, to tyrosine (Tyr), the product. Decreased PAH activity results in Phe accumulation, called hyperphenylalaninemia. Phenylalanemia causes neurotoxicity and causes mental retardation. More than five hundred mutations in genes coding for PAH have been determined, resulting in PAH activity ranging from severe inhibition, when PAH is as low as 5% of normal, to mild PKU when PAH is near normal.[9] More than half of children with PKU have one of the milder phenotypes.[10]

Neonates are screened for this disorder at birth, and it has an incidence of one in ten thousand. Phenylalanine is found in all protein foods, and neonates diagnosed with this condition are placed on a phenylalanine-restricted diet and supplemented with tyrosine, vitamins, minerals, and other amino acids. Milk, cheese, egg, meat, and fish are typically omitted or greatly restricted in diets for those with PKU, not because they are disproportionately high in Phe alone, but because they are disproportionately high in protein and therefore, disproportionately high in most amino acids, including Phe. Vegetables and cereal grains are often emphasized in PKU diets, even though they are protein-containing foods, because they are relatively low in Phe. While effective, maintaining this severely limited diet is quite difficult in school-age children, leads to socially awkward situations for adults, and is complicated in pregnant women.

Since 1999 several clinical trials have reported positive results in restoring the activity of PAH and reducing serum Phe by providing high doses tetrahydrobiopterin (BH_4), a PAH cofactor, to restore the K(m) of PAH. In one small study, serum Phe concentrations declined in four of five children with a loading dose of 10 mg BH_4 per kg/body weight.[11]

Table 1.1. Milestones in Medical Biochemistry

1902, Archibald E. Garrod, MD
1913, Michaelis-Menten equation created
1953, Watson and Crick discovered double-helix of DNA
1990s, Bruce Ames, PhD at UC Berkeley, discovered genetic changes alter the Michaelis-Menten equation and *are correctable*
1984–2008, biochemical testing perfected

A larger, twelve-month study conducted in from December 2000 through December 2002 stratified thirty-eight children into three groups: mild hyperphenylalaninemia (pre-treatment plasma phenylalanine less than 600 µmol/L, N = 10, age fifteen days to ten years), mild PKU (pre-treatment plasma phenylalanine 600–1200 µmol/L, N = 21, age eight days to seventeen years), and "classic" or severe PKU (pre-treatment plasma phenylalanine greater than 1200 µmol/L, N = 7, age one day to nine years).[10] Participants consumed a meal containing 100 mg Phe per kg/body weight loading dose, followed one hour later with 20 mg BH_4 per kg/body weight. Blood Phe levels were determined at baseline, before BH_4, and at four, eight, and fifteen hours after BH_4. A child whose Phe level decreased by more than 30% after BH_4, compared with levels observed after the Phe loading test, was considered responsive to therapy. All children classified as having mild hyperphenylalaninemia and seventeen of the twenty-one children (87%) with mild PKU responded to BH_4 treatment. Among responders, the decrease in Phe ranged from 37 to 92%.

These studies indicate that infants and children with this disorder should now also be tested for their responsiveness to BH_4 therapy, as it may allow many of them to consume a less-restrictive diet, and some to even cease the therapeutic diet altogether. Additionally, this research demonstrates that even in "severe" genetic conditions, there may be some enzyme activity that can be stimulated with pharmacologic dosages of nutrients, and that diseases once viewed as incurable may in fact be ameliorated with nutrients. See Table 1.1 for an overview of historical landmarks in the development of medical biochemistry.

Functional Biochemical Testing Versus Genetic Testing

Our functional biochemical testing approach contrasts sharply with the genetics-only model of testing and treatment in that testing for a gene does not provide sufficient data to understand how the gene is affecting the physiology of the body. Only by testing the underlying biochemical pathways can one delineate the multivariate determinants of health and disease.

In 1953 James Watson, PhD, and Francis Crick, PhD, unveiled their double-helix model of DNA.[12] On the day of their breakthrough, Dr. Watson walked into an English pub and announced they had "found the secret of life."[13] Their work revolutionized how scientists, physicians, and the general public view biology, and massive efforts were subsequently launched to decode the human genome. After1990, almost a half century after Drs. Watson and Crick's discovery, the U.S. Department of Energy and the National Institutes of Health coordinated the Human Genome Project. The project finished in 2003 after successfully sequencing the three billion base pairs of the human genetic code. Yet, despite the vast amount of data both these milestones yielded, in many respects Dr. Watson's statement was naive.

In 2009 the *Journal of the American Medical Association* (*JAMA*) published a three-part series reviewing current genetic testing technologies, their clinical applications and utility.[14-16] These articles defined the standards by which laboratories, clinicians and policymakers measure the validity, reliability and applications of genetic testing.

There are several fundamental premises underlying genetic testing. One is the Hardy-Weinberg equilibrium (HWE), which states that both allele and genotype frequencies in a population are constant and that there is no population-wide variation in frequencies from generation to generation unless specific disturbing influences are introduced. This concept is appropriate and accurate in a closely controlled environment, such as a laboratory. However, in the real world, the HWE does not apply. Research in population genetics shows that allelic variation, or "genetic drift," occurs and is the norm. Therefore, the associations between genotypes and diseases, although possibly appropriate in limited circumstances today, will be different and cumulative between generations.

Second, and perhaps as important, is that the genome-wide associations yield false-positive and false-negative results that are higher than in traditional medical studies. In effect, the results of genetic testing bear little resemblance to the actual risk for disease expression. According to a 2008 article in *JAMA* that evaluated the usefulness of direct-to-consumer personal genome testing, "A statistically significant association between a particular genomic variant and a disease dose not necessarily mean that the presence of the variant in a given individual is clinically meaningful. Many of variants discovered in genome-wide association studies are associated with only marginal increases in risk, with odds ratios often 1.5 or less. The usefulness of this information for clinical decision making is unclear."[17]

In fact, with genetic testing, physicians end up spending the limited and precious time they have with patients explaining the tests instead providing other more helpful information and treatments. The authors go on to state, "…the time spent following up on [genetic testing] with patients detracts from time spent on other activities more relevant to the health of the patient. Worse, it could result in a cascade effect, in which ambiguous, incidental, or false-positive results lead to further workup that creates anxiety, cost and potential harm."

Additionally, the genetics approach in effect freezes the mindset of the clinician into a very narrow spectrum of diagnosis and potential treatments. The clinician is then forced to admit that there is very little he or she can do once there is a genetic loading for a disease, even if that loading is a false-positive. But more importantly, they are unaware that there are ways to manipulate the biochemical expression of the alleles.

The genome is, indeed, the blueprint for biological life; however, post-translational modifications of amino-acid sequences create many more proteins than the genes coding them. A surprising finding of the Human Genome Project is that there are far fewer protein-coding genes in the human genome than there are proteins (thirty to forty thousand protein-coding genes[18] vs. approximately five hundred thousand proteins, respectively[19]). Disease is not expressed at the level of the gene but at the level of the basic biochemical pathways. This creates a biochemical phenotype, which can change based on the subcellular miroenvironment, or what is called epigenetics.

Billions of dollars of private and public monies have flowed into genetic testing research that is based on a false paradigm that in most cases is not clinically relevant. Healthcare spending by the present administration of President Barack Obama continues to emphasize genetic testing, which is a paradigm based on false premises, that will not yield the promised benefits.

Unlike genetic testing, functional biochemical testing is a multivariate analysis that evaluates complex biochemical pathway functions and outcomes. It does so by virtue of reporting at the level of substrates, cofactors, and products in biochemical pathways. These data are then used to construct the biochemical pathways in an individual patient to determine where the problem is in the pathway and how that is reflected in different types of symptoms and diseases.

The authors have extrapolated these biochemical determinants into the Neustadt-Pieczenik Postulates.

Neustadt-Pieczenik Postulates:

1. Genetics explains no more than 25% of disease expression.
2. The Law of Parsimony should be strictly followed in clinical diagnoses; that is, use the simplest explanation to describe the suite of presenting symptoms.
3. Symptoms and diseases are biochemical in nature, not primarily genetic, which can be altered by dietary, lifestyle and environmental factors.
4. Biochemistry is simply how the body uses amino acids, vitamins, minerals, and fats to do its job, and how infections, environmental toxins (e.g., toxic metals, solvents), and allergies interfere with optimal biochemical function to cause symptoms and diseases.

5. If a person was not sick last year or last month, and he or she is sick now, then something's changed in his or her biochemistry.

6. Through sophisticated functional biochemical testing, the underlying causes of multiple symptoms and diseases can be analyzed simultaneously and quickly corrected to promote health.

7. Modifications of biochemical functioning using targeted therapies require clinicians be specifically trained to properly conceptualize, interpret and apply this multivariate approach to dynamic physiological processes.

8. This approach can be curative.

The concept and clinical application of providing customized treatments based on this biochemical testing is *the* major concept that underlies functional biochemical testing and the subsequent treatment approaches, all of which is based on pure science, clinical trials, and more than one hundred years of medical observations and experimentation. More often than not, treatments based on biochemical testing are correcting the specific problems that contribute directly to the patient's symptoms and diseases. At the same time clinicians skilled in this paradigm can evaluate the data to predict future diseases and symptoms, which can also be corrected to prevent future disease expression. No genetic testing can accomplish the multiplicity of tasks that this functional biochemical approach can do.

At the same time, the cost of the test and treatments are much less than genetic testing, CT scans, MRIs, PET scans and invasive procedures, which people frequently undergo before discovering functional biochemical medicine. The functional biochemical approach is an exponential value-added one. Multiple cases in this book illustrate how people routinely spend tens of thousands of dollars on standard tests and procedures before being evaluated by Dr. Neustadt. The clinical benefits obtained through functional testing and treatment modalities cost a fraction of the conventional approaches that provided no benefits.

An example of this testing has been applied to correct mature onset asthma, which was resistant to the classical treatments of antibiotics, steroids, and a bronchodilator inhaler. In this particular case, the underlying cause of the patient's asthma was a block in the conversion of phenylalanine to epinephrine and norepinephrine (Figure 1.7). Epinephrine is a bronchodilator, and without it pulmonary constriction occurs. This concept is not commonly understood in medicine, but it has powerful implications. In this case, the patient spent more than fifteen thousand dollars on pulmonary and cardiac stress testing and medications, without any benefit. Indeed, this approach caused considerable suffering.

Figure 1.7. Pathway and factors for conversion of phenylalanine to epinephrine

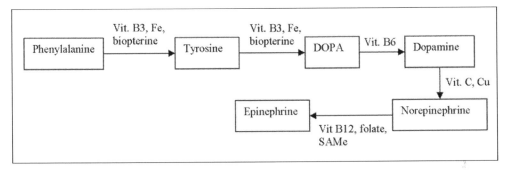

Abbreviations: Vit. B3 = Vitamin B3 (niacin); Fe = iron; Vit. B6 = Vitamin B6 (pyridoxine); Vit. C = Vitamin C; Cu = Copper; SAMe = S-adenosylmethionine

In this case, the patient's functional biochemical testing revealed the underlying causes of the mature onset asthma. The test showed elevated serum tyrosine, low erythrocyte copper, low urinary vanilmandelate (a marker for norepinephrine and epinephrine), and functionally low B-complex vitamins as indicated by elevated urinary alpha-ketoisovalerate (Table 1.2). These functional biochemical markers were treated by providing a customized program to effectively push the pathway in the direction of health, and the patient's asthma resolved.

Table 1.2. Test results for a sixty-two-year-old male with mature onset asthma

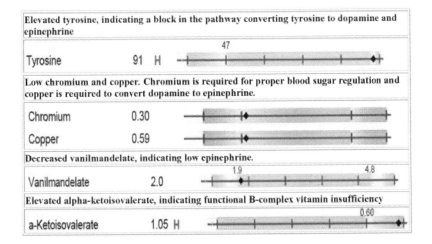

Application to Single Nucleotide Polymorphisms

This field of study has been applied to less severe forms of genetic variations known as single nucleotide polymorphisms (SNPs). A SNP is defined as a change in a gene that appears in more than 1% of the population, which suggests a pattern of inheritability rather than chance alone.[20] Additionally, at least one-third of all SNPs alter the binding affinity for an enzyme and its substrate.[3] When this occurs, providing higher dosages of the cofactors necessary for enzyme function can help restore enzyme activity and essentially force the enzyme reaction in the desired direction.[3]

A common example is the SNP for the methylene tetrahydrofolate reductase (MTHFR) enzyme. This enzyme is responsible for activating folic acid so that it can function to decrease homocysteine, a protein that, in epidemiological studies, has been shown to increase the risk for cardiovascular disease, osteoporosis, cancer (colorectal, lung, cervical), and dementia.[21-27] In vitro evidence suggests that homocysteine may be a causative factor in these diseases through three distinct mechanisms: 1) It directly damages DNA by causing fragmentation in a way that mimics radiation exposure. 2) It directly damages the endothelium and causes a decrease in oxygen and nutrient delivery to tissues including heart, brain, and bone. 3) It decreases nitric oxide (NO), an important signaling molecule in the body that plays a role in blood vessel dilatation and neurotransmission.[28]

A relatively common genetic alteration in the gene coding for MTHFR is the *C677T* autosomal recessive mutation. Heterozygotes for this mutation exhibit a 30% reduction and homozygotes a 65% reduction in enzyme activity compared with normozygotes.[20] That is, the enzymes created by the different MTHFR SNPs, such as the C→*T* polymorphism, require higher amounts of folic acid to function. These polymorphisms occur in up to 50% of Caucasians, 47% of Koreans, 42% of Hispanics, 29% of Native Americans, 12% of African-Americans, and 10% of Asian Indians.[20]

The result is that people with the MTHFR *C→T* polymorphism may have higher concentrations of homocysteine due to a decreased ability to utilize folic acid. The deleterious effects of this genetic polymorphism can be overcome simply by providing higher dosages of folic acid, as has been demonstrated in dose-response studies.[29, 30]

However, just because someone has this genetic polymorphism doesn't mean that it's elevating his or her homocysteine level and that a patient requires higher doses of folic acid.

High doses of folic acid may actually be harmful if not needed. Large doses of folic acid given to an individual with an undiagnosed vitamin B12 deficiency could correct megaloblastic anemia without correcting the underlying vitamin B12 deficiency, leaving the individual at risk of developing irreversible neurologic damage.

Instead of merely testing the MTHFR genetic polymorphism, which is what genetic testing companies are doing, clinicians must instead be testing for homocysteine and *functional deficiencies* in folic acid as indicated by an elevated urinary formiminoglutamate. Genetic testing companies can test MTHFR and homocysteine, but it is more expensive than simply testing homocysteine and urinary formiminoglutamate.

The other major issue here is that homocysteine may be elevated not just with a functional folic acid deficiency, but may also be elevated with deficiencies in vitamins B12 or vitamin B6. Therefore, the *only* and *best* way to determine what specific nutrient(s) someone needs to lower his or her homocysteine, is to test urinary formiminoglutamate, urinary xanthurenate (or urinary kynurenate), and urinary methylmalonic acid (MMA). The data generated by these tests provide an unparalleled snapshot into how the body is functioning instead of a static picture of the genes, which may not actually be expressed and may not actually be impacting health.

Importantly, Dr. Neustadt recently had a patient who came to him who had previously been tested for the MTHFR genetic polymorphism. This patient tested positive for the MTHFR polymorphism and her doctor, without testing homocysteine, put her on high doses of folic acid. She ended up leaving that doctor because she moved to a new town and had stopped all the doctor's recommendations months before coming to see Dr. Neustadt. Dr. Neustadt ordered her previous labs from her old doctor and confirmed the MTHFR diagnosis. However, Dr. Neustadt then tested her homocysteine (plasma homocysteine), and it was not elevated. She did not need to be taking high doses of folic acid, which is what these genetic testing companies are recommending based on their myopic genetic paradigm.

As previously mentioned, in addition to genetics, an enzyme's requirement for nutrients can increase in response to hormones secreted during physical and psychological stress, lack of exercise, poor diet, and free radical damage related to the aging process. As people age, nongenetic factors (e.g., diet and lifestyle) play more important roles in the development of diseases than do genetics. In the vast majority of situations, genetics merely predispose someone to a disease, but lifestyle and nutritional status determine whether that disease actually develops. A decreased ability to utilize nutrients can be overcome in many instances by giving higher dosages of the nutrient. This forces biological reactions to go in the desired direction and helps reverse the deleterious effects of aging and other stressors.

This fundamental concept has revolutionary implications for medicine. Medicine often looks at genetic alterations in their extreme forms (e.g., Down's syndrome and Marfan syndrome). However, much more common are subtle functional changes in biochemistry caused by genetic individuality, nutritional status, and lifestyle that do not cause readily apparent physical or mental abnormalities. Instead, the changes in biochemical function are more insidious, and the resultant diseases do not appear until later in life.

Liver Detoxification Pathways and Breast Cancer

Liver detoxification pathways serve as excellent examples of an organ-specific genetic expression that exert powerful control over the development, maintenance, and progression of diseases. For example, liver detoxification pathways greatly influence the risk for and development of cancers.

Metabolism of endogenous and exogenous compounds occurs in the liver via two major complementary pathways called phase I and phase II. These two phases work in sequence, with most metabolites of phase I passing through phase II. Phase I enzymes are a super-family of hemoproteins called cytochrome P450s (CYP) enzymes. They oxidize relatively nonpolar molecules, increasing their polarity and allowing them to be excreted in the urine. The main CYP isoforms are 1A2, 1B1, 2D6, 2C9, 2C19, and 3A4.[31-33] Phase II enzymes catalyze conjugation reactions to compounds, such as glutathione, that facilitate elimination.[20] Phase II enzymes include glutathione *S*-transferases, UDP-glucoronosyl-transferases, *N*-acetyltransferases, microsomal epoxide hydrolase, and sulfotransferases.[34]

Decreased activities of phase II enzymes are associated with the pathogenesis of diseases. Overexpression of the CYP1B1 isoform has been associated with the development of numerous cancers, including prostate, breast, and ovarian cancers, as well as serous and mucinous carcinomas, but its overexpression is not detected in normal tissues.[35-39]

Estrogen is predominantly metabolized in the liver via two pathways. One pathway produces 2-hydroxyestrogen (2-OHE). The other first metabolizes estrogen to 4-hydroxyestrogen (4-

OHE), then to 16-hydroxyestrogen (16-OHE). The 2-OHE is metabolized via the CYP1A system, while 4-OHE is metabolized via the CYP1B1 pathway.

The exact concentrations of these estrogen metabolites don't appear to be as important as the ratio of the metabolites. A 2-OHE:16-OHE ratio (called a 2:16 OHE) less than 1.8 is associated with increased risk of breast cancer.[40] Increasing this ratio may decrease a woman's risk of developing breast and uterine cancer. In one epidemiological study, a decrease in breast cancer risk of 45% was seen in the highest quintile of 2:16-OHE compared to the first quintile.[40] The 2-OHE pathway is *inducible*, meaning that its activity can be increased so that 2-OHE production is increased. This can be accomplished by consuming higher amounts of cruciferous vegetables such as broccoli and cauliflower, and also by taking a dietary supplement containing adequate amounts of diindolylmethane (DIM). In a pilot study, administration of 108 mg DIM daily increased the 2:16-OHE ratio in postmenopausal women by 47% (from 1.46 to 2.14), which approached statistical significance (P=.059).[41] This study provides another good illustration of how a person's unique biochemistry can be modulated to affect disease risk.

Heal the Gut, Heal the Body

One morning Dr. Pieczenik received a phone call from a friend, a woman in her late fifties. She called about other matters, but the conversation turned to health. She asked one important question that Drs. Neustadt and Pieczenik hear all the time. She and her husband were lying in bed talking the night before about their own health, visits to doctors, symptoms, and the many medications, including pills and injections, that they'd been prescribed by different physicians. This is very common—people go to different specialists for their problems, but there is no one doctor coordinating their care who can evaluate their health medically and holistically.

So they asked Dr. Pieczenik the question, "What are we putting into our bodies and what are we doing to ourselves? We are not getting better." They were concerned about the effects of too many medications on their bodies and weren't sure why they were taking them. Moreover, their doctors had basically prescribed one medication after another without ever telling them how long they would be taking the medicines. One by one, pills were added that they would be taking indefinitely. No plan, logic or rationale was ever given to them as to how the doctors were going to restore their health. Instead, these two people were experiencing what too many people have been living with for years—being totally confused as to what was happening to them.

Dr. Pieczenik explained to them that with some of their diagnoses, such as rheumatoid arthritis, the fundamental dysfunction may have actually started in the gut. Allopathic physicians are not taught this. So the notion that any disease entity except specific and overt gastrointestinal disorders could be related to the gut is completely alien to allopathic physicians.

In contrast, a fundamental approach to health in naturopathic medicine is to "treat the gut." Approximately 80% of all immune proteins are produced in the gut.[42] The immune tissue in the gut is called Gut-Associated Lymph Tissue (GALT) and is the largest immune organ in the body.[43] This makes sense when you begin thinking functionally. What's the role of the immune system? Very simply, it protects you from the outside world—bacteria, viruses, and parasites. What part of your body is most exposed to the outside world? Most people intuitively would say their skin, but in fact it's your intestines (stomach, small, and large intestines). The intestines have a surface area that's 3,229 to 4,306 ft². That's 20% of a football field![44] (An American football field has a surface area of 21,600 ft².)

Technically the intestines are outside the body. They form a hollow tube from mouth to anus. When people put food or drink in their mouths, it doesn't actually enter their bodies until it is absorbed through the cells lining the gut. The intestine's exposure to the outside world and all of its dangerous microbes is inspiring. Every day the average person consumes three to five pounds of food.[44] That's three to five pounds of the outside world being ingested. And every piece of food contains potentially millions of organisms, both harmful and beneficial.

Even when someone eats optimally, he or she may not be digesting and assimilating the nutrients properly. There are three major reasons for this: digestion may not be functioning properly due to chronic stress; food intolerances may be causing chronic immune activation in the gut;[45-47] or intestinal bacterial, fungal, or protozoal infections, called *intestinal dysbiosis*,[45, 48] may be causing inflammation and decreased digestion. Each of these situations can occur individually or together, placing one at risk for decreased ability to digest and absorb nutrients.

Digestion involves the breakdown of large molecules into smaller, readily absorbed molecules. Whereas some digestion begins with the production of enzymes in the mouth, the stomach is where the process of digestion really takes place. Cells in the stomach excrete specific enzymes to break apart fats, starches, and proteins. The enzymes, however, are inactive and must be activated by stomach acid. When someone produces enough stomach acid, proper digestion in the stomach occurs. But many people don't produce enough stomach acid. Low stomach acid production is called *hypochlorhydria,* and when no stomach acid is produced, it's called *achlorhydria.* Decreased stomach acid production occurs from aging, caffeine, overeating, stress, medications (especially those that block the production or excretion of stomach acid such as Protonix, Tagamet, Pepcid, Axid, Zantac, Prevacid, Prilosec, Aciphex, and Nexium), alcohol, and stomach surgeries that destroy the acid-producing cells.

Many people produce less stomach acid as they age. It's been estimated that 10–21% of people sixty to sixty-nine years old, 31% of those seventy to seventy-nine years old, and 37% of those above the age of eighty have hypochlorhydria or achlorhydria, and this rate may be higher in people with autoimmune conditions.[49, 50] One question posed to patients to screen for their risk of low stomach acid is, "Do you feel fuller sooner than you used to and stay full longer than you used to when you eat?" If the answer is yes, it may be that they have low stomach acid, since decreased stomach acid increases the amount of time food sits in the stomach before passing into the small intestines. When stomach acid is low, vitamins and minerals may not be efficiently released from the food that contains them.

This may result in decreased availability of nutrients for absorption and nutritional deficiencies. People with low stomach acid have been shown to be at increased risk for vitamin and mineral deficiencies.[51-55] Symptoms of low stomach acid production include bloating or distension after eating, diarrhea or constipation, flatulence after a meal, hair loss in women, heartburn, indigestion, malaise, and a prolonged sense of fullness after eating.[55, 56] Additionally, the risk of hip fracture increases by 22% after one year and nearly 60% after four years in people taking proton-pump inhibitor (e.g., Protonix, Prilosec, Nexium, Aciphex) and H2-receptor antagonist (H2-blockers; e.g., Cimetidine and Ranitidine (Zantac)) medications compared to people not taking them.[57]

Stomach acid plays two other important roles. It acts to sterilize food and signals the lower esophageal sphincter (the muscle separating the esophagus from the stomach) to close.[58-60]

When low stomach acid production decreases the ability of the lower esophageal sphincter to close, the result is that the acid produced in the stomach can reflux up into the esophagus and cause symptoms of GERD.[61] The typical medical response to gastric reflux, which can cause burning, coughing, and asthma-like symptoms, is to prescribe acid-blocking medications.

However, the actual cause in many people is too little acid and not too much acid.[61] Decreased acid production can occur as a result of decreased histidine, an amino acid that is required for acid secretion.[62] This amino acid is tested as part of an amino acid blood panel, which may diagnose the underlying cause in some patients. Stomach acid production can also be tested by using a meter, called a Heidelburg pH capsule test. Providing histidine to people with low stomach acid can improve their stomach acid production. Low stomach acid can also occur in from infections, such as *Helicobacter pylori* (*H. pylori*) in the stomach.[61] Additionally, when people have low stomach acid production, some doctors provide hydrochloric acid capsules for people to take with meals that help improve their digestion and eliminate GERD. There are some instances when people should not supplement with acid pills, and the authors of this book strongly advise people against supplementing with hydrochloric acid unless under the care of a doctor.

The gut normally contains about four hundred different species of bacteria, which are required for normal digestion and absorption of nutrients.[63, 64] It has been estimated that there are more bacterial cells in the gut than all the cells in the body combined.[65] These beneficial bacteria are required for normal digestion and absorption of nutrients. When inadequate sterilization of food occurs, however, pathogenic bacteria, viruses, and fungi can pass into the small intestines. This disrupts the healthy ecology in the gut and alters the delicate balance between healthy and unhealthy microbes.

It is now recognized that gut immunity plays a central role in systemic health. For example, it has been observed that gastric acid suppression, using H_2-blockers and proton pump inhibitors is associated with an increased risk of community-acquired pneumonia. It is suspected that acid suppression results in insufficient elimination of pathogenic organisms. It has therefore been suggested that patients at higher risk of pneumonia should only be prescribed proton pump inhibitors at lower doses and only when necessary.[66]

Dysbiosis can occur with the overgrowth of pathogenic bacteria, parasites and/or fungi. Symptoms of intestinal dysbiosis include abdominal gas and bloating, post-nasal drip, "brain fog" (feeling like you're just not mentally sharp), and sugar cravings.[67] Abdominal gas and bloating are caused by fermentation of food by microorganisms, which produce methane.

Post-nasal drip is caused by immune system activation in the gut. GALT activation stimulates histamine release, which increases vascular permeability and causes symptoms of rhinitis or post-nasal drip. Sugar is the preferred energy source for the fungi, which can lead to sugar cravings. Bacteria and fungi secrete their own waste products, such as ammonia, that can enter the blood stream, cross into the brain, and cause brain fog. Additionally, intestinal bacterial overgrowth is now understood to be a risk factor for developing gastroesophageal reflux disorder (GERD).[68]

The new generation of stool tests is the most sensitive and specific at detecting gut pathogens. Normally when physicians suspect a parasitic infection an *ova & parasite (O&Px3)* test is ordered. In an O&Px3 test, a patient provides samples of his or her stool that are evaluated under a microscope by a parasitologist who is literally looking for small parasite eggs or the mature parasites themselves. To detect a parasite the parasitologist must rely not just on his or her skills, but also on luck. The parasitologist must be lucky enough to have a stool sample by chance that had a large enough parasite or egg in it to be seen through a microscope. They do not look at every square centimeter of the stool but take samples from the stool to look at. They therefore must also be lucky that the random sample they took had something in it. This test is highly unreliable.

The most advanced testing analyzes stool samples for parasite DNA fragments. Instead, the stool sample is run through a sophisticated machine. The stool sample does not need to have an intact parasite or egg in it. This eliminates the role of luck in the process. Instead, the stool sample is run through a sophisticated machine and only five cells from an organism are required to detect it. Common parasite infections diagnosed by this technology include hookworm (*Necator americanus*), whipworm (*Trichuris* sp.), and *Cryptosporidium* sp.

Additionally, from this one stool sample the tests can detect *H. pylori* infection in the stomach, bacterial and yeast infections in the intestines, and if your intestines are low in healthy bacteria. *H. pylori* is a bacterium that colonizes the stomach and is considered a Type I carcinogen. Most physicians will not test for any of these other infections, even though the symptoms significantly overlap with a parasite.

Parasitic diagnoses are very rare because most physicians are not trained in parasitology. It's the rare medical school that will expose its students to a six- or eight-week course in parasitology. Most standard medical evaluations do not include a parasite test, and even when they do it's an extremely insensitive test. Why might it be important to test for parasites? Because the symptoms mimic many other diseases. For a list of symptoms that can be caused by parasites, see Table 1.3.

Food intolerances can also cause decreased absorption of nutrients by creating chronic inflammation in the intestines. Eighty percent of the immune system is clustered around the intestines.[42] When people repeatedly consume food that causes an immune activation in the gut, it creates intestinal irritation.[69] Over time, the cells lining the intestines become damaged. This can create malabsorption with decreased ability to assimilate nutrients from food. An extreme example of this is Celiac disease. Intolerance to wheat, rye, barley, and oats characterizes this disease. The immune system actually reacts to gluten contained in these foods. This causes intestinal inflammation and destruction of the cells lining the intestines. Celiac disease has wide-ranging symptoms, including fatigue, anemia, joint pains, depression, loss of balance, and malnutrition.[70, 71]

More frequently, people will react to foods that they crave, such as milk and eggs, which can be detected through a special blood test. This blood test is called an IgG food intolerance test, and

Table 1.3. Symptoms of parasite infections

| All skin problems |
| Anal itching (especially at night) |
| Anemia |
| Any menstrual complaint |
| Arthritic pains |
| Bed wetting |
| Burning in the stomach |
| Chronic candida |
| Chronic fatigue |
| Chronic sinus or ear infections |
| Chronic viral syndromes |
| Constipation |
| Crawling feeling under the skin |
| Cysts and fibroids |
| Depression |
| Diarrhea |
| Digestive problems |
| Drooling while sleeping |
| Eating more and still being hungry |
| Floaters |
| Forgetfulness |
| Gas and bloating |
| Hemorrhoids |
| Inability to gain or lose weight |
| Irritable bowel syndrome |
| Itchy ears or nose |
| Liver/gallbladder trouble |
| Mucous in stools |
| Numb hands |
| Pain in the back (thighs or shoulders) |
| Pain in the navel |
| Prostate problems |
| Sexual dysfunction in men |
| Urinary tract infections |
| Water retention (mostly from tapeworms) |
| Yeast infections |

people with rheumatoid arthritis, eczema, and other conditions have been shown to have elevated IgG antibodies to foods.[72, 73] IgG is a protein produced by the immune system. Most doctors only test for IgE-mediated allergies, which are also called "immediate hypersensitivity reactions." An IgE-mediated-immune response is responsible for the life-threatening reaction in some people to bee stings or peanuts. IgG, on the other hand, is a delayed-type-hypersensitivity reaction that, as the name implies, is not immediately apparent.[74] People who test negative on an IgE test can be positive on an IgG test.[75]

IgG reactions may take hours or days to appear, and symptoms can include post-nasal drip, gas and bloating, difficulty losing weight, joint aches, eczema, fatigue, and others. Food intolerances can cause these diverse symptoms for various reasons. Similar to bacterial and fungal dysbiosis, the immune-system activation caused by food intolerances can cause post-nasal drip. Gas and bloating is a result of incomplete digestion of food and the resultant fermentation of these food particles by microorganisms in the intestines. Difficulty losing weight may result from an increased cortisol response by the body due to the continual stress placed on the immune system. When cortisol is chronically elevated, it causes an accumulation of abdominal fat.

The explanation for eczema and joint pains is a little more complicated. When the immune system in the intestines is activated, the antibody-antigen complexes enter the blood stream. An antibody is the protein produced by the immune system such as IgG, and an antigen is the molecule against which the immune system is reacting, such as a protein in milk. These antibody-antigen complexes travel from the intestines to the liver, where they are broken down for elimination by the body. This process is like a conveyor belt where the antibody-antigen complexes are delivered to the liver for processing, but the amount of complexes delivered to the liver over time can overwhelm the liver's ability to detoxify them.

When this occurs, the complexes pass through the liver and enter the systemic circulation. Like bits of sand in a river, these complexes can settle out of the blood stream where the flow of blood slows down. This occurs in the skin and joints. When these complexes are deposited in skin and joints, they act as irritants that can create local immune-system activation and produce such symptoms as joint pains and eczema. Frequently, the joint pains will be migratory, meaning different joints will be affected at different times.

Chronic stress predisposes people to low stomach acid production and food intolerances.

This is because stress stimulates the release of cortisol, norepinephrine, and epinephrine. These are part of the *flight or flight* response to stress. The analogy that's often used to teach this concept to medical student is, "Imagine that you're being chased by a tiger." The body has two responses. It either flees or battles it out. In either case, cortisol and epinephrine are secreted to prepare people for action. They increase blood flow to skeletal muscles and decrease it to the intestines. These hormones also increase heart rate and alter blood flow in the brain. By shifting blood flow away from the intestines and to the muscles, digestion decreases. This can also cause damage to the cells lining the intestines and create a "hyperpermeable gut." When digestion decreases, it allows larger food particles to enter the small intestines, where food is absorbed through the lining of the gut and into the body. The larger food particles, combined with the damaged lining of the gut, can activate the immune system and create food intolerances.

As the reader now might understand, many health complaints are directly related to and caused by an unhealthy intestinal tract. Identifying any food allergies and intestinal infections are crucial to healing the gut. The goal is remove the things (e.g., aggravating foods and infections) that are causing the problems and then initiate a gut repair protocol using specific nutrients to make the gut healthy. One key nutrient is L-Glutamine, an amino acid that is an energy source for cells in your digestive tract. This provides nutrition to the gut to help the cells heal. Herbs that soothe the gut are also sometimes used.

The ability of the body to catabolize toxins and excrete them in the urine and stool is a vital determinant for overall health. While as much as 75% of detoxification activity occurs in the liver, much of the remainder takes place in the intestinal mucosa wall. Still, an additional small percentage occurs in other tissues. Although we usually think of the liver as the detoxification site, it makes sense that the intestine also plays an important role in detoxification, since the gastrointestinal lining provides the initial physical barrier to the largest load of xenobiotics, including orally ingested drugs.

The GI tract has indeed developed a complex physical and biochemical system to manage this load, as evidenced by the high concentration of detoxification enzymes present in the tip of the villi,[76, 77] by the antiporter activity and b the P-glycoprotein (Pgp) system. Pgp is a membrane-bound, adenosine triphosphate (ATP)-dependent efflux pump that moves substrates out of cells.[78] It can reduce the therapeutic effect of drugs by increasing their excretion.[79] Pgp upregulation by cancer cells and bacteria decreases the amount of drugs that can accumulate in the cells and results in resistance (multi-drug resistance, MDR).

The GI tract also influences detoxification by hosting gut microflora capable of producing compounds that may either induce or inhibit detoxification.[80, 81] Although the liver and intestinal mucosa contain the majority of the detoxification enzymes, the importance of detoxification explains the occurrence to some degree of detoxification activity in all cells.

Chapter Two

MD versus ND

The reason Drs. Neustadt and Pieczenik wrote this book was to elucidate the types of diseases that can be treated in what is considered an alternative way as opposed to a strictly allopathic approach. This book is not intended to denigrate any part of the allopathic system, but the principles annunciated in this book are quite simple—that allopathic medicine has either forgotten or purposely hijacked the financial and educational elements of medicine that were extant long before the pharmaceutical industry became a prominent and, the authors believe, a largely destructive force in medicine.

The fundamental philosophical and operational difference between allopathic (conventional) medicine and integrative medicine, as practiced by naturopathic physicians and integrative medical doctors, is that allopathic medicine *suis generis* treats primarily symptoms. It is a disease model of care that looks at symptoms as distinct entities to be treated. In contrast, integrative medicine does not simply focus on treating individual symptoms of disease but rather looks at the person and asks, "Why is this person sick, and what is keeping the patient from being well?" This is a crucial distinction.

The next time you go see your physician, ask him or her (if he or she give you the time to do so), "What is your philosophy of medicine?" and "What is the definition of health?" All medicine, business, and life choices stem from a basic philosophy. The philosophy of the dominant medical system today is one of treating symptoms with drugs and surgery, even though they may not be required and good, scientifically based evidence supports other, more effective methods. What is meant by "good, scientifically based evidence"? This is a large question that gets into the field of study called epistemology, which means how we know what we know. In medicine the answer comes through probability and statistical data. It also comes from having financing available to conduct the ostensibly objective studies that hospitals, insurance companies, nurses and doctors use to justify their treatments.

The reality is, however, that 80% of clinical decisions are not based on the randomized, double-blind, placebo-controlled trial, which is the gold standard for research. Instead, it's based on "consensus"; that is, whatever other doctors are doing. This translates legally into the definition of the "standard of care" in medicine. The standard of care is simply what the other doctors in a given geographic area are doing. For example, the standard of care in treating depression is to prescribe an anti-depressant medication such as Paxil or Prozac. The doctors who are prescribing this, and the teaching physicians in the medical colleges who are advocating the use of these medicines, are receiving their information from the FDA and the pharmaceutical sales representatives.

However, a January 17, 2008, report from the *New England Journal of Medicine* (NEJM) titled, "Selective Publication of Antidepressant Trials and Its Influence on Apparent Efficacy" revealed that the effectiveness of a dozen popular antidepressant medications has been seriously exaggerated by selective publication of favorable results.[82] Consequently, doctors and patients have gotten a distorted view of the usefulness of antidepressants like Effexor, Zoloft, Welbutrin, Paxil, and Prozac.

The researchers reviewed seventy-four studies registered with the FDA between 1987 and 2004. These clinical trials involved twelve antidepressants and 12,564 patients. All but one of the thirty-eight studies reporting positive results was published. The other thirty-six studies reported negative or questionable results, and twenty-two of those studies were never published. Of the fourteen that were published, the researchers said that at least eleven of these studies mischaracterized the results and presented a negative study as "positive." The bottom line according the researchers was that "the studies the FDA judged as positive were approximately twelve times as likely to be published in a way that agreed with the FDA analysis as were studies with nonpositive results."

For example, researchers discovered that five trials on the effectiveness of Zoloft were submitted to the FDA. The drug appeared to work better than the placebo in two of them; however, in three other trials, the placebo did just as well at reducing the symptoms of depression. But only the two favorable studies were published, and Pfizer, who manufactures Zoloft, discusses only the positive results in Zoloft's literature for doctors.

What Pfizer, the FDA, and other major drug companies (Wyeth, Schering-Plough, GlaxoSmithKline, Eli Lilly, and Forest) have done is to ignore the negative findings of studies when the results go against their corporate interests. Their unethical and dangerous behavior results in drugs being approved that have only questionable effectiveness while minimizing the serious consequences of their side effects.

According to the researchers, these biases inflated the reported effectiveness of all twelve of the antidepressant medications studied that were approved between 1987 and 2004. These medications are Zoloft, Serzone, Remeron, Welbutrin SR, Paxil, Cymbalta, Effexor, Effexor XR, Celexa, Lexapro, Prozac, and Paxil CR.

This skews the medical profession's understanding of how effective a drug is for a particular condition. It is especially significant in the evolving movement called "evidence-based medicine," which depends heavily on the analyses of published studies to make treatment decisions. And it places physicians in an exceedingly awkward position, since we strive to make the best choices for our patients based on published research.

After analyzing all of the data, the researchers of the NEJM study determined that antidepressant medications really only work 40 to 50% of the time. The data was so blatantly biased that the effectiveness of these medications was artificially inflated by nearly 70% in the case of Serzone and by 64% in the case of Zoloft.

This blatant distortion of data to meet the bottom-line goals of pharmaceutical companies is similar to the tobacco industry, which sat on research that showed nicotine was addictive. Several pharmaceutical companies have already been sued over this matter by the New York State Attorney General. Just like the tobacco companies did, the pharmaceutical companies continue to deny any wrongdoing.

What should patients do? If symptoms of depression don't seem to improve, it may not be the patient that's the problem, it may be the drug. Other medications may be helpful, as may alternative therapies such as nutritional medicine, exercise, and certain botanicals.

In addition to selectively publishing results, many studies have concluded that the marketing tactics of providing gifts and trips to physicians effectively buys the doctor's compliance and agreement to prescribe the medications. GlaxoSmithKline spent more than $500 million over two years paying physicians to give lectures, sponsoring events, and sending attractive women pharmaceutical representatives out into the field to create a demand for their new drug for restless leg syndrome (RLS), called Mirapex (Pramipexole Dihydrochloride).

From a business perspective, since the general public can only get these products from their doctors, the pharmaceutical industry views medical offices as distribution channels and doctors as sales people for their products, just as toy stores are distribution channels for toy companies. And they demand patients ask their doctors about the drugs. This approach has been wildly successful. GlaxoSmithKline brought in more than $3 billion in revenues for Mirapex. Unfortunatel, RLS is a newly-created disease that was promoted to create revenue for a new drug for a company that was stagnant and looking for new revenue streams. In short, RLS is a questionable disease, Mirapex is a questionable treatment, and GlaxoSmithKline's, funding of marketing for this disease is a clear conflict of interest—all hallmarks of disease mongering at its finest.

Make no mistake, the authors are entrepreneurs who believe in making honest products for a decent profit for real and existing problems. Creating new problems and paying physicians to promote them under the guise of objectivity is repugnant, especially when the Hippocratic code of ethics in medicine states, "Above all else do no harm."

And much harm is perpetrated on the unwitting doctors who are too busy to read the primary studies and the naive public. Most doctors are very decent people who are overworked and underpaid. The result is a medical system that is totally out of control. While it is trying to do good, it is unfortunately doing much harm (Table 2.1).

Table 2.1. Frightening Facts from Major Medical Journals2–5

One hundred and eighty thousand people die each year partly as a result of injury caused by the very medical procedure or drug that was supposed to help the patient. Over the course of a year, that's the equivalent of three jumbo jet crashes every two days.
Twenty million antibiotic prescriptions are written every year for viral infections, which antibiotics cannot treat
7.5 million unnecessary medical procedures are performed each year

17% of all hospital admissions are caused by the side effects of drugs
Prescription drug-related diseases and death cost the US $77 billion dollars annually
20% of all patients admitted to a university hospital suffered iatrogenic injury. 36% of those admitted to a teaching hospital suffered an iatrogenic event, of which 25% were serious or life threatening.
64% of cardiac arrests at a teaching hospital were preventable. Most were due to use of medications.
198,815 people are killed each year by medications
8.8 million people are hospitalized each year because of medications
28% of all hospital admissions are caused by medications, which costs as much as $182 billion dollars
51% of approved drugs have serious side effects not detected before marketing approval

Another example is in the field of psychiatry. A July 12, 2008, article in the *New York Times* highlighted the fact that money from pharmaceutical companies is tainting clinical judgment in the field of psychiatry. Specifically, Senator Charles E. Grassley, a Republican from Iowa, demanded that the American Psychiatric Association (APA), the field's premier professional organization, give an accounting of its financing. The association is the official voice of the psychiatric establishment. It publishes the field's major journals and its standard diagnostic manual, the Diagnostic and Statistical Manual of Mental Disorders, 4th Edition (DSM-IV).

It appears that the financial influence of the pharmaceutical industry has shaped the practice of this nonprofit organization that reports to be independent in its viewpoints and actions. It recently came to light that the chairman of the department of psychiatry at Stanford University and the top physician and president-elect of the APA, Dr. Alan F. Schatzberg, has $4.8 million in stock holdings in a drug development company. Dr. Schatzberg also had to disclose his more than six figures in consulting fees, grants, and pension funds, all funded by pharmaceutical companies promoting their own narrow financial agendas.

In 2006 the drug industry accounted for the APA's $62.5 million in financing. About half of that money went to drug advertisement in psychiatric journals and exhibits at the annual meeting. And the other half went to sponsoring fellowships, conferences, and industry symposiums at the annual meeting. Not only did the APA subsequently clear Dr. Schatzberg of any ethical conflicts, but he was then anointed president of the association.

If that isn't evidence enough, let's go back to RLS. The Restless Leg Foundation was founded in 2005. Its budget at that time was $1.4 million, and 44.8% of that revenue came from companies that manufacture RLS drugs.

In a 2005 ground-breaking article published in the *Public Library of Science*, Drs. Steven Woloshin and Lisa M. Schwartz from the Veterans Affairs Outcome Group and Dartmouth Medical School defined the strategies of "disease mongering."[83] According to these researchers. "*Disease mongering* is the effort by pharmaceutical companies (or others with similar financial interests) to enlarge the market for a treatment by convincing people that they are sick and need medical intervention. Typically, the disease is vague, with nonspecific symptoms spanning a broad spectrum of severity—from everyday experiences many people would not even call symptoms, to profound suffering. The market for treatment gets enlarged in two ways: by narrowing the definition of health so normal experiences get labeled as pathologic, and by expanding the definition of disease to include earlier, milder, and presymptomatic forms (e.g., regarding a risk factor such as high cholesterol as a disease in itself)."

Regarding cholesterol, readers should know that more than 50% of first heart attacks occur in people with normal cholesterol, and in fact, there is no hard evidence to confirm that lowering cholesterol in and of itself reduces the risk of a first heart attack. There is good evidence, however, that if you have had a heart attack, cholesterol-lowering medication may help prevent a second one from occurring. However, the pharmaceutical industry's voracious appetite for new customers is now extending to the very young. A Policy Statement by the American Academy of Pediatrics (AAP) advocates prescribing cholesterol-lowering medications in children as young as ten years old.[84] This opens up a huge new market for the pharmaceutical industry, despite the fact that there are no (repeat, no) clinical trials proving the safety of these medications in children or whether medicating children this young prevents future coronary artery disease, the stated goal of cholesterol-lowering therapies.

Woloshin and Schwartz go on in their article to succinctly define how drug companies manipulate the public. Pharmaceutical companies promote diseases and drugs through four different channels:

1. "Disease awareness" campaigns
2. Direct-to-consumer drug advertising
3. Funding of disease advocacy groups, usually under the cover of nonprofit organizations.
4. Providing pre-written stories to harried journalists who are overworked and do not have the time or the scientific background to adequately evaluate the veracity of the information they're being fed.

Drug companies also practice *disease mongering* by:

1. Exaggerating the prevalence of disease
2. Encouraging more diagnosis of the disease
3. Suggesting that all disease should be treated

These companies also underestimate the risks of treatment. For example, Mirapex can cause uncontrollable sexual urges and compulsive gambling in users. There may indeed be people who suffer painful RLS and may benefit from medications or other approaches; however, Drs. Neustadt and Pieczenik strongly believe that the disease mongering of the drug industry has caused people to be overdiagnosed, misdiagnosed, overmedicated, and undertreated for their true problems (see RLS cases).

Journalists are unwittingly selling sickness, much like the physicians who are prescribing antidepressant medications and thinking they are using the most evidence-based, cutting-edge scientific approach to helping their patients, when they have in fact over-sold the product. Physicians, journalists, and the general public are literally the victims of a very sophisticated media campaign by the pharmaceutical companies who have high-powered marketing and PR firms, lobbyists, and doctors on their payrolls to be their hired guns.

This is no different from psychological warfare tactics, in which Dr. Pieczenik is an internationally recognized expert. Dr. Pieczenik was a principal architect of the strategy to take down the Soviet Union in the 1980s and 1990s during the Reagan and Bush Sr. administrations. The principles of denial, distraction, and distortion are all the basic elements used in psychological warfare. It is also called "PsyWar." The same tactics used in PsyWar are used by the pharmaceutical and advertising industries to persuade and propagandize physicians and consumers to think and behave in the way that benefits the narrow financial interests of the drug companies.

Despite the drug industry's monumental efforts to convince the public that their intentions are benign and their products are all good, the news for the pharmaceutical industry has been very bad lately. An August 2007 study published in the *Journal of the American Geriatrics Society* concludes that people who use the H2-blocker medications that block stomach acid, which include Zantac, and Tagamet, have a nearly 250% increased risk of dementia.[85] Just a few months earlier, in May 2007, the U.S. Food and Drug Administration (FDA) issued a warning for the diabetes medication, Avandia, which was shown to increase the risk of heart attacks by 30 to 40%,[86] and in 2006 *JAMA* reported that the risk of hip fracture increases by 22% after one year and nearly 60% after four years in people taking proton-pump inhibitors, another class of stomach acid-blocking medications that includes Prilosec, Nexium, Protonix, Aciphex and Prevacid.[57] These revelations are just the surface of a very serious problem in the American health care system that are putting millions of people at risk.

This story of medications causing dangerous, sometimes fatal, adverse effects is not new. Another *JAMA* study in 1998 concluded that fatal drug reactions for hospital patients "appear to be between the fourth and sixth leading cause of death," and that the rate of fatal drug reactions had been stable for the past thirty years, killing more than one hundred thousand people annually. Drs. Neustadt and Pieczenik don't want to give the impression that they condemn pharmaceuticals; however, the data are clear. Medications can be very dangerous as well as very helpful. One has to always balance out the potential risks with the potential benefits, and that discussion should always be between patients and their physicians.

It's not even that pharmaceuticals per se are the culprit, but it's the underlying paradigm in medicine that needs to be changed. The current philosophy underlying medicine today is that diagnoses are based on symptoms and treated with medications to simply suppress the symptoms instead of identifying and treating the underlying causes of disease. For example, depression is treated conventionally by prescribing antidepressant medications, which, while they may be very helpful, do nothing to correct the underlying biochemical causes of the depression. Taking Prozac may lift someone's mood and help him or her through a difficult period, but no one has a deficiency in Prozac.

In contrast, a medical system that approaches diseases by first evaluating the underlying biochemical causes of the disease and then correcting them using targeted biochemical therapies can correct the underlying causes. The biochemical pathways for depression are well documented. Without being too complicated, the mood-lifting hormone serotonin is produced in the body by transforming the amino acid tryptophan into serotonin, and requires vitamin B6 and magnesium to do so. There are other relevant pathways for generating mood and energy, but this simple example illustrates a central point about the underlying biochemical dynamics of depression.

The concept of causality versus symptoms is a major shift in paradigm, which the pharmaceutical companies and the medical profession in general have not accepted. The premises for this new biochemical medicine are simple. *Premise 1:* health and disease are biochemical; *Premise 2:* if someone was healthy and he or she is not now, something's changed in his or her biochemistry; *Premise 3:* if you identify and treat the underlying biochemical dysfunction(s), disease may be prevented and cured.

Dr. Pieczenik's case is a perfect example. Several years ago he was diagnosed with mature-onset asthma, for which he was prescribed steroids and an inhaler. He refused to take these medications because he knew that they would cause their own adverse effects. Instead, he made an appointment with Dr. Neustadt, who ordered a comprehensive biochemical screen that tested more than 450 variables of biochemical function. Biochemical testing revealed the underlying cause for Dr. Pieczenik's asthma. His symptoms resulted from an inability to produce the hormone epinephrine, which is a bronchodilator, because he became deficient in copper, which is required to convert the amino acid tyrosine to epinephrine. Within two weeks of starting the therapy to realign his copper, all of his breathing difficulties stopped, and he has had no breathing problem since then. Essentially, his incurable disease was cured.

The problems with the pharmaceutical industry and our current medical system stem from an inherently incorrect philosophy where symptoms are treated and not their causes, and medical testing does not evaluate the underlying biochemical causes of disease.

In contrast, Naturopathic Medicine stems from a basic philosophy that is fundamentally different from conventional, allopathic medicine. Naturopathic doctors are physicians clinically trained in natural and integrative therapeutics and whose philosophy is derived in part from a Hippocratic teaching more than two thousand years old: *Vis mediatrix naturae*—nature is the healer of all diseases.

Their practice is based on the same basic biomedical science foundation that allopathic practice utilizes; however, their philosophies and approaches differ considerably from their conventional counterparts.

When a patient comes to see Dr. Neustadt for the first time, he always starts the appointment by asking the patient, "We're meeting each other for the first time, so I'm wondering if you have any questions for me about naturopathic medicine or how I approach medicine." Frequently patients will be unfamiliar with naturopathic medicine but will have made an appointment because they'd been through the conventional medical system without any relief or even with their health worsening. But more importantly, they are frequently frustrated that they'd spent so much time and money with physicians and still did not have any answers as to why they were sick.

New patients will often ask, "What is naturopathic medicine?" Dr. Neustadt answers, "Naturopathic medicine is different from allopathic medicine by its philosophy. No matter what you do in life—business, sports, parenting—the way you act is determined by the fundamental philosophy that informs what you do. There are six philosophical tenets of naturopathic medicine (Table 2.2). The fist tenet is First Do No Harm, which is the same as allopathic physicians. However, the way that it's applied is very different between conventional and naturopathic medicine. Allopathic physicians are trained almost exclusively in drugs and surgery. And they do an excellent job with those modalities. However, naturopathic physicians, while trained in drugs and minor surgery, and can prescribe medications in many states in which they're licensed, stress other modalities, such as nutritional medicine, botanical medicine, physical medicine (chiropractic-type adjustments, hot and cold therapies), lifestyle counseling, homeopathy and dietary counseling.

"The second philosophical tenet is called the Healing Power of Nature. This is a belief that there are inherent systems in the body that strive to maintain homeostasis and keep you healthy. For example, when you cut yourself you tend to heal naturally, without any assistance. I have interpreted this based on my special interests in botany, nutritional medicine, and biochemistry to emphasize specific testing methods that identify the underlying biochemical causes of disease, which can often be corrected quickly by providing the properties the body needs to heal. The ultimate goal of all of this is tied into the third philosophical tenet of naturopathic medicine, which is to Treat the Cause. In contrast, allopathic medicine by and large only treats symptoms and does not identify or correct the underlying causes of disease.

"Doctor as Teacher is the next philosophical tenet. It's important for me to spend time educating my patients about their own bodies and health so that they can take better care of themselves, so that hopefully they do not need to be dependent on doctors or medicines. However, doing this takes time. That's why first appointments, except for acute situations like an upper respiratory infection, are scheduled for a minimum of forty-five minutes to an hour. I simply cannot get enough information about a patient and practice the best possible medicine I can in less time. A ten- or fifteen-minute first appointment is simply not long enough. This extra also allows me to learn about my patients so that I can Treat the Whole Person, which is the next philosophical tenet in naturopathic medicine.

"The last philosophical tenet is Prevention. That is, the best medicine not only treats what you have wrong now but also prevents future diseases. That's why nutritional medicine is so important. Since nutrients are used in every body system, optimizing nutritional status results in 'side benefits.' These are therapeutic benefits beyond what we're just trying to treat at any given time. For example, muscle cramps can be caused by low magnesium. Providing extra magnesium can cure these muscle cramps, but may also play a role in preventing cardiovascular disease."

"There are four nationally accredited naturopathic medical schools in the United States. Prerequisites for these schools are nearly identical to those of conventional, allopathic medical schools. The first two years of education are also nearly identical. Naturopathic medical students have to take anatomy, histology, biochemistry, pathology, physiology, embryology, and other courses. However, in addition to those classes, we also have courses in naturopathic medical philosophy and survey courses in Ayurvedic and Traditional Chinese Medicine. Not that we practice these forms of medicine, but it educates us to be aware of other philosophies of medicine and when it might be helpful to refer to one of these other practitioners. After two years of school, just like our allopathic colleagues, naturopathic medical students take national basic sciences board exams. After the fourth year and completion of the clinical coursework, we take our national clinical board exams for licensure.

Table 2.2. Philosophical tenets of Naturopathic Medicine

Naturopathic Philosophy	Definition
First Do No Harm —primum non nocere	Naturopathic medicine stresses using therapies that are safe and effective.
The Healing Power of Nature —vis medicatrix naturae	The human body possesses the inherent ability to restore health. The physician's role is to facilitate this process.
Discover and Treat the Cause, Not Just the Effect —tolle causam	Physicians seek and treat the underlying cause of a disease. The origin of disease is removed or treated so the patient can recover.
Treat the Whole Person —tolle totum	The multiple factors in health and disease are considered while treating the whole person. Physicians provide flexible treatment programs to meet individual health care needs.
The Physician is a Teacher —docere	The physician's major role is to educate, empower, and motivate patients to take responsibility for their own health. Creating a healthy cooperative relationship with the patient has a strong therapeutic value.
Prevention Is the Best "Cure"	Naturopathic physicians are preventive medicine specialists. Physicians assess patient risk factors and heredity susceptibility and intervene appropriately to reduce risk and prevent illness. Prevention of disease is best accomplished through education and a lifestyle that supports health.

The implementation of the naturopathic medical philosophy is based on what's called, The Therapeutic Order (Table 2.3). This encourages doctors to use the most appropriate intervention to create the greatest benefit with the least amount of harm. For example, lifestyle changes, stress reduction, and nutritional interventions are safer and can be more effective at times than reaching straight for the prescription pad to prescribe a drug. However, the Therapeutic Order stresses that if one needs a medication or surgery immediately, then that's what should be prescribed, but there are more options to consider than just drugs and surgery.

Table 2.3. The Therapeutic Order

Therapeutic Order	Definition
Stimulate the *Vis Medicatrix Naturae*	This is the force that moves us toward health; it is the *essence* that invigorates us. Some modalities utilized to stimulate the "Vis" include hydrotherapy, exercise, yoga, meditation, nutritional medicine. and botanicals.
Tonify weakened systems	Specific organs and body systems are sometimes over or underexpressed by people differently. For example some patients may have a hyper- and hypo-stimulated immune system, nervous system, endocrine system, cardiovascular system, etc.
Correct structural integrity	Disease may affect all systems if the communication pathways are compromised by spinal and nervous systems mal-alignment.
Prescribe specific, pathology-based, natural substances	This is often necessary in more advanced pathology. However, this is done while addressing the underlying imbalance. When patients are in severe distress or pain and they need relief immediately, naturopathic physicians may prescribe medicines, which allow for symptom palliation or cure in the case of antibiotics for bacterial infections.
Pharmacological agents for pathology	There are many situations that warrant conventional medical treatments and therapies. In these cases, naturopaths utilize allopathic medicine as a subset to our modalities.

Surgery, suppressive drugs, radiation, and chemotherapy	These interventions save lives and help many, many patients to live longer, happier, healthier lives. As Dr. John Bastyr said toward the end of his retirement, "Do what works." Many patients continue to lead healthy lives thanks to these interventions.

In conclusion, what we propose to do is give you a group of patient cases that were examined and treated by Dr. John Neustadt in his clinic. After all identifying patient information was removed from these cases, Dr. Pieczenik evaluated them to discuss how the conventional medical approach would intersect with Dr. Neustadt's naturopathic approach. We hope you enjoy this journey. It has been a challenging opportunity for both doctors. Please understand that neither wishes to denigrate the other's approach to medicine, but rather wants to juxtapose these approaches for readers so that they may appreciate the how these two fields may eventually be joined to form a truly integrative and health-oriented national medical system.

Chapter Three

Functional Biochemical Testing in Clinical Practice

This type of testing is so sophisticated the authors have called it a "Metabolic CT Scan," abbreviated MetaCT™. Like a CT scan, it provides an unparalleled view into the body. However, unlike a CT scan, which is static, the MetaCT test is dynamic and provides information about how the body is actually functioning. Additionally, it does not require expensive equipment or the exposure to dangerous X-rays. The most comprehensive of the MetaCT tests is the MetaCT 400, which requires eight vials of blood, one vial of urine and a stool sample. It reports more than 450 NBI Analytes™ (Table 3.1). Each of the sections of the MetaCT 400 test can be broken down and ordered as individual tests.

Table 3.1. List of NBI Analytes on the MetaCT 400 Test

Complete Blood Count with Differential	White Blood Cells (WBC), Red Blood Cells (RBC), Hemoglobin, Hematocrit, Mean Corpuscular Volume (MCV), Mean Corpuscular Hemoglobin (MCH), Mean Corpuscular Hemoglobin Content (MCHC), Red Cell Distribution Width (RDW), Platelets, Neutrophils, Lymphocytes, Mid Cells

Serum Chemistries	Fasting Blood Glucose, Urea Nitrogen (BUN), Creatinine, Total Protein, Albumin, Total Bilirubin, Calcium, Sodium, Potassium, Chloride, Carbon Dioxide, Carbon Dioxide, Alkaline Phosphatase, SGOT (AST), SGPT (ALT)
Vitamins	Coenzyme Q10, 25-Hydroxyvitamin D, Alpha-Tocopherol, Gamma-Tocopherol, Vitamin A, Beta-Carotene
Intracellular Essential Minerals	Calcium, Chromium, Copper, Magnesium, Manganese, Potassium, Selenium, Zinc
Toxic Metals	Aluminum, Arsenic, Cadmium, Lead, Mercury
Iron Panel	Serum Iron, Iron Binding Capacity, % Saturation, Serum Ferritin
Lipid Panel	Total Cholesterol, Triglycerides, HDL Cholesterol, LDL Cholesterol, Cholesterol-to-HDL Ratio, Lipoprotein(a)
Thyroid Panel	Thyroid Stimulating Hormone (TSH), Total T3, Free T4
Gastrointestinal Microbiology Profile	Bacteria infections: Helicobacter Pylori (H. pylori), Clostridium difficile., E. coli, Campylobacter spp., Aeromonas spp. and others Fungal infections (e.g., Candida sp.) Parasitic infections (e.g., Giardia lamblia, Cryptosporidia spp.) Healthy gut bacteria: Bacteroides sp., Clostridia sp., Prevotella sp., Fusobacteria sp., Streptomyces sp., Mycoplasma sp., Lactobacillus sp., Bifidobacter sp.

Amino Acids	**Essential Amino Acids (EAA):** Arginine, Histidine, Isoleucine, Leucine, Lysine, Methionine, Phenylalanine, Threonine, Tryptophan, Valine **EAA Derivatives—Neuroendocrine Metabolism:** Gamma-Aminobutyric Acid, Glycine, Serine, Taurine, Tyrosine **EAA Derivatives—Ammonia/Energy Metabolism:** Alpha-Aminoadipic Acid, Asparagine, Aspartic Acid, Citrulline, Glutamic Acid, Glutamine, Ornithine **Sulfur Metabolism:** Cystine, Cytathionine, Homcysteine **Additional Metabolites:** Alpha-Amino-N-Butyric Acid, Alanine, Anserine, Beta-Alanine, Beta-Aminoisobutyric Acid, Carnosine, Ethanolamine, Homocysteine, Hydroxylysine, Hydroxyproline, 1-Methylhistidine, 3-Methylhistidine, Phosphoethanolamine, Phosphoserine, Proline, Sarcosine
Markers of Free Radical Damage	Lipid peroxides, 8-Hydroxy-2'deoxyguanosine, p-Hydroxyphenyllactate (HPLA)
Markers of Inflammation	Ferritin, Fibrinogen, High Sensitivity C-Reactive Protein (hsCRP), Quinolinate

Hormones and Neurotransmitter Markers	Insulin, Testosterone, Sex Hormone Binding Globulin (SHBG), Free Androgen Index (calc.), Vanilmandelate, Homovanillate, 5-Hydroxyindoleacetate, Kynurenate. **Optional test:** Urinary estrogen ratio (risk factor for breast and cervical cancers)
Fatty Acid Profile	<u>Polyunsaturated Omega-3</u>: Alpha-Linolenic Acid (ALA), Eicosapentaenoic Acid (EPA), Dosapentaenoic Acid, Docosahexaenoic Acid (DHA) <u>Polyunsaturated Omega-6</u>: Linoleic Acid, Gamma Linolenic Acid (GLA), Eicosadienoic Acid, Dihomogamma Linolenic Acid (DGLA), Arachidonic Acid (AA), Docosadienoic Acid, Docosatetraenoic Acid <u>Polyunsaturated Omega-9</u>: Mead Acid <u>Monounsaturated</u>: Myristoleic Acid, Palmitoleic Acid, Vaccenic Acid, Oleic Acid, 11-Eicosaenoic Acid, Erucic Acid, Nervonic Acid <u>Saturated</u>: Capric Acid, Lauric Acid, Myristic Acid, Palmitic Acid, Stearic Acid, Arachidic Acid, Behenic Acid, Lignoceric Acid, Hexacosanoic Acid <u>Odd Chain</u>: Pentadecanoic Acid, Heptadecanoic Acid, Nonadecanoic Acid, Heneicosanoic Acid <u>Trans Fatty Acids</u>: Palmitelaidic Acid, Total C:18 Trans <u>Ratios (Calculated)</u>: LA/DGLA, EPA/DGLA, AA/EPA, Triene/Tetraene

Urinary Organic Acids	<u>Fatty Acid Metabolism</u>: Adipate, Suberate, Ethylmalonate
	<u>Carbohydrate Metabolism</u>: Pyruvate, Lactate, Beta-Hydroxybutyrate
	<u>Energy Production (Citric Acid Cycle)</u>: Citrate, cis-Aconitate, Isocitrate, Alpha-Ketoglutarate, Succinate, Fumarate, Malate, Hydroxymethylglutarate
	<u>B-Complex Vitamin Markers</u>: Alpha-Ketoisovalerate, Alpha-Ketoisocaproate, Alpha-Keto-Beta-Methylvalarate, Xanthurenate, Beta-Hydroxyisovalerate
	<u>Methylation Cofactor Markers</u>: Methylmalonate, Formiminoglutamate
	<u>Detoxification Indicators</u>: 2-Methylhippurate, Orotate, Glucarate, Alpha-Hydroxybutyrate, Pyroglutamate, Sulfate

IgG 90-Food Allergy Panel	Almond, Apple, Apricot, Asparagus, Aspergillus mold, Avocado, Banana, Barley, String Bean, Beef, Black pepper, Blueberry, Broccoli, Cabbage, Cantaloupe, Carrot, Casein, Cashew, Cauliflower, Celery, Chicken, Chocolate, Cinnamon, Clam, Coconut, Codfish, Coffee, Corn, Crab, Cranberry, Cucumber, Egg White, Egg yolk, Flounder, Garlic, Ginger, Grape, Grapefruit, Halibut, Honeydew, Lamb, Lemon, Lentil, Lettuce, Lima Bean, Lobster, Mackerel, Malt, Milk, Mushroom, Mustard Greens, Navy Bean, Oat, Olive, Onion, Orange, Oyster, Green Pea, Peach, Peanut, Pear, Pecan, Green Pepper, Pineapple, Pinto Bean, Pistachio, Pork, Potato, Rice, Rye, Salmon, Sesame, Shrimp, Soybean, Spinach, Strawberry, Sunflower, Sweet Potato, Tea, Tomato, Trout, Tuna, Turkey, Vanilla, Watermelon, Walnut, Wheat, Baker's Yeast, Brewer's Yeast, Zucchini **Optional Additional Tests:** Celiac Disease Panel; IgE food and environmental allergies panel.

From the test report, skilled clinicians can derive a patient's risk factors for diseases and symptoms. They can determine the likelihood that a person is suffering from specific symptoms, such as depression and gas/bloating, without ever even having to see the patient. This is similar to a radiologist reading a CT scan on a computer screen a thousand miles away from the hospital where the patient is. From these NBI Analytes, a table of risk factors can be created (Table 3.2).

Table 3.2. Summary of Risk Factors

Categories	Analytes
Fatigue and depression	Allergies to dairy and eggs, low ferritin, low omega-3 fatty acids, low amino acids, decreased ability to utilize nutrients for energy production, low-normal B12 and other B-complex vitamins.
Anxiety	Low glycine
Decreased strength	Low essential amino acids
Gas/Bloating	Moderate and severe food allergies to milk and eggs; intestinal bacterial overgrowth.
Cancer risk	Low vitamin D2 (breast, colorectal, cervical); elevated glutamic acid-to-glutamine ratio; elevated free radical damage to DNA
Cardiovascular disease risk	High cholesterol, low omega-3 fatty acid and fatty acid ratios, low vitamin D2, elevated lipid peroxides
Dementia	Functional vitamin B12 deficiency, elevated 8-Hydroxy-2-deoxyguanosine
Toxic exposure	Elevated urinary pyroglutamate, 2-Methylhippurate, and glucarate. Elevated whole blood arsenic and mercury.
Decreased ability to lose weight	Food allergies, low essential fatty acids, low amino acids, inability to utilize nutrients for cellular energy

Chapter Four

Gastroenteritis

Gastroenteritis is an inflammation of the gastric mucosa. It can occur anywhere in the gastrointestinal tract. There are two major categories of gastroenteritis: acute and chronic. Acute gastroenteritis may be caused by an acute infection which might be self-limiting, such as a mild food poisoning. The major risk with an acute gastroenteritis is dehydration and electrolyte depletion secondary to diarrhea and vomiting.

This section of the book does not discuss acute gastroenteritis because it is not as relevant to the functional biochemical approach as are the more chronic conditions. Acute gastroenteritis can be a medical emergency and is more of a triage situation where the patient might needs to be quickly stabilized. In these cases, the conventional medical approach is superior.

Chronic gastroenteritis, like many chronic conditions, tends to be multifactorial, and includes infectious gastroenteritis, irritable bowel syndrome (IBS), Crohn's disease and ulcerative colitis (UC). Many times people suffer for years with chronic gastroenteritis. They have been to multiple doctors, including their primary care physician, gastroenterologist, and psychiatrists. They are often referred to psychiatrists or simply prescribed antidepressants because depression frequently accompanies chronic gastroenteritis. The conventional approach is unable to diagnose and fix the underlying causes.

One caveat is that Dr. Neustadt does not have much experience working up and treating Crohn's disease and UC by the medical biochemistry approach. Therefore, the authors do not know how effective this approach would be for these conditions. On the other hand, Dr. Neutadt has charted a more than 80% success rate at working up and successfully treating patients with IBS and infectious gastroenteritis using this approach.

Dr. Pieczenik

In the old days we used to do barium contrast tests to rule out ulcers and tumors, and these procedures are still done. However, more modern techniques, such as colonoscopies, are more frequently ordered. Today even a virtual colonoscopy exists whereby the patient merely swallows a telemetry capsule that transmits images of the GI tract as it passes through.

If it's not an obvious infectious disease or irritable bowel disease (IBD), or if upon ordering an O&Px3 the test come back negative for parasites, then symptomatic treatment is all that can be offered. In particular, physicians might prescribe antispasmodics, antiprotazoals, antidepressants, anti-inflammatories, and analgesics.

The notion that there might be underlying biochemical causes of chronic gastroenteritis is alien to the conventional medical community, as is the fact that the bowels are the largest immune organ in the body. In turn, all we monitored was the CBC, serum chemistries, blood pressure and temperatures, as well as a few specialized tests to rule out pancreatitis and other conditions. If infections were suspected, we would have ordered a stool test to see if we might be able to culture out any organisms. Equally important, medical doctors do not appreciate the grave consequences hyperpermeable gut can have on systemic health.

Dr. Neustadt

There are many documented causes of chronic gastroenteritis, and the conventional approach is very effective in many cases. However, the conventional medical community has been completely unaware of the functional determinants of gastrointestinal health and disease, including healthful gut flora and IgG-mediated food allergies. Additionally, the wider medical community is not using the most up-to-date testing methodology for diagnosing infections, which uses DNA probes. This testing approach is more sensitive and specific than the classical O&Px3, which has many false negatives. Finally, chronic gastroenteritis can lead to malabsorption syndrome, which in turn can cause many subsequent biochemical abnormalities and symptoms such as depression, anxiety, headaches, rashes, and thyroid dysfunction.

Case: Infectious Gastroenteritis in a Fifty-one-year-old Woman

This case demonstrates several difficulties when trying to fit this new approach into a classic diagnostic category.

The patient, a fifty-one-year-old woman, had been suffering for thirteen years with severe abdominal pain. She was originally diagnosed with endometriosis and subsequently had a radical hysterectomy. However, her abdominal pain continued unabated. Not surprisingly, an O&Px3 was ordered and came back negative. When she came to the clinic she was taking Paxil 20 mg daily for depression and Percocet multiple times each day for chronic, daily lower left abdominal pain and cramping.

The pain occurred daily and was so severe she rated the pain a ten out of ten, with ten being worst. At her first appointment with Dr. Neustadt she mentioned suffering with sudden-onset diarrhea for the previous five days. She had no appetite and had barely been eating during this period. She appeared completely exhausted and pale. Dr. Neustadt concluded that this was an emergency. He immediately put her on a rehydration intravenous drip with supportive vitamins and minerals. By the time she left his office her energy had increased and her color returned to normal. He instructed her to purchase Imodium at the drug store, which she did, as a symptomatic treatment to stop the diarrhea. However, even when the diarrhea stopped her pain and gas and bloating continued.

She had a colonoscopy within the past two years. She reported that in the lower left quadrant the gastroenterologist found some "irritated" tissue and told her that this was "endometriosis." This patient also reported that she had been a competitive swimmer in high school and was a runner-up to the U.S. Olympic Swim Team. She had completely deteriorated since her days as a competitive athelete to the point that she was in constant pain, depressed, and overweight.

After Dr. Neustadt reviewed her medical history and symptoms with her, it became quickly apparent that endometriosis was not the current problem. In fact, Dr. Neustadt suspected that at least since the time of her hysterectomy she had been misdiagnosed. Dr. Neustadt came to this conclusion because the pain from endometriosis tends to be cyclical and flares up just before menses. But she no longer produced endogenous hormones or had menstrual cycles because both of her ovaries had been removed.

Dr. Neustadt suspected that undiagnosed severe food allergies and intestinal infections would be causing her problems. The fact that she had been a competitive athlete and that she had no appetite placed her in a high risk category for nutritional deficiencies.

Her MetaCT 400 test results showed:

Food allergies			
Egg, White	1,036	Severe	+5
Egg, Yolk	661	Mod	+4
Intestinal Bacterial Infections			
Bacillus sp.		2.9E+008	H
Citrobacter sp.		1.9E+009	H
Pseudomonas sp.		2.0E+008	H
Salmonella sp.		4.3E+008	H
Intestinal Yeast Infection			
Yeast/Fungi; taxonomy unavailable.		+1 => 100 pg DNA/g specimen	
Intestinal Parasite Infection			
Necator americanus (hookworm)		Positive	

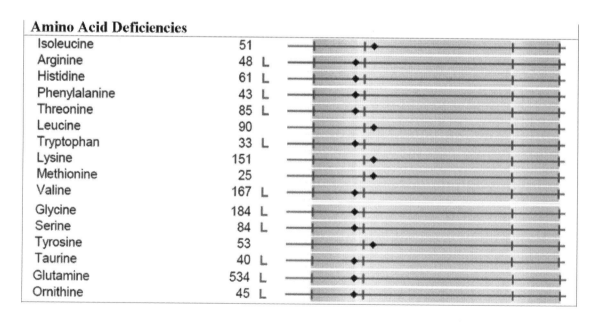

Amino Acid Deficiencies

Isoleucine	51	
Arginine	48	L
Histidine	61	L
Phenylalanine	43	L
Threonine	85	L
Leucine	90	
Tryptophan	33	L
Lysine	151	
Methionine	25	
Valine	167	L
Glycine	184	L
Serine	84	L
Tyrosine	53	
Taurine	40	L
Glutamine	534	L
Ornithine	45	L

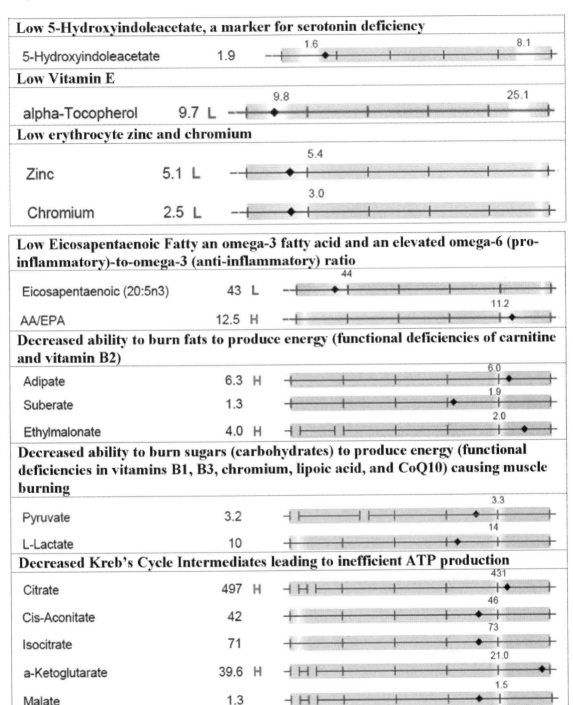

Low 5-Hydroxyindoleacetate, a marker for serotonin deficiency

5-Hydroxyindoleacetate   1.9

Low Vitamin E

alpha-Tocopherol   9.7 L

Low erythrocyte zinc and chromium

Zinc   5.1 L

Chromium   2.5 L

Low Eicosapentaenoic Fatty an omega-3 fatty acid and an elevated omega-6 (pro-inflammatory)-to-omega-3 (anti-inflammatory) ratio

Eicosapentaenoic (20:5n3)   43 L

AA/EPA   12.5 H

Decreased ability to burn fats to produce energy (functional deficiencies of carnitine and vitamin B2)

Adipate   6.3 H

Suberate   1.3

Ethylmalonate   4.0 H

Decreased ability to burn sugars (carbohydrates) to produce energy (functional deficiencies in vitamins B1, B3, chromium, lipoic acid, and CoQ10) causing muscle burning

Pyruvate   3.2

L-Lactate   10

Decreased Kreb's Cycle Intermediates leading to inefficient ATP production

Citrate   497 H

Cis-Aconitate   42

Isocitrate   71

a-Ketoglutarate   39.6 H

Malate   1.3

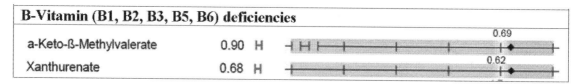

B-Vitamin (B1, B2, B3, B5, B6) deficiencies		
a-Keto-ß-Methylvalerate	0.90 H	0.69
Xanthurenate	0.68 H	0.62

Upon hearing the results of her testing, the patient cried because she finally had an explanation for her years of suffering, and even better, she now had hope. The approach to her treatment was a multifaceted integrative approach. It's important for readers to understand that medications are necessary when they're needed, but they are completely overused in our society. Here's her treatment plan, which ultimately had completely cured her.

Treatment Plan

Diet:

AVOID all eggs and all egg-containing products for eight weeks, and then reintroduce them into your diet. See the handout on egg allergies.

For hookworm infection:

Rx Mebendazole 100 mg orally twice daily for three days (90% effective).

ACTIVATED CHARCOAL: Take two capsules after eating lunch and two capsules two hours later; repeat with and after dinner. Take for one month and then discontinue.

IMMUNOPRO: Take one scoop twice daily in room-temperature water or a non-acidic juice (e.g., apple juice, grape juice).

For bacterial infection
(***Do not start until after finishing Mebendazole treatment***):
Rx Ciprofloxacin 500 mg orally twice daily for seven days

BERBERINE FORTE: Take one capsule twice daily with food.

ENTEROPRO: Take one capsule daily with food. Keep refrigerated.

For fungal infection
(***Start this at the same time as the Ciprofloxacin treatment***):

Rx Nystatin 500,000 units orally twice daily for three months.

* * *

Do not start the remainder of the program until the Ciprofloxacin is finished

For amino acids (Note: You may mix all the amino acid powders together):

RESCULPT: Stir or blend two (2) scoops (23g) of ReSculpt into 8 fl. oz. of water, milk, or juice once daily.

GLYCINE POWDER: Mix a half teaspoon daily with water with or between meals. Take one bottle of this and then discontinue.

GLUTAMINE RX: Mix one teaspoon twice daily in water and drink.

TAURINE POWDER: Take half teaspoon daily. Take one bottle of this and then discontinue.

PERFUSIA SR: Take two capsules twice daily. Take two bottles and then discontinue.

For extra zinc and chromium:
PROMINERALS: Take three capsules daily with food. Take two bottles and then discontinue.

For omega-3 fatty acids:
CARLSON'S COD LIVER OIL: Take one tablespoon (equivalent of three teaspoons) daily. Keep refrigerated.

For ability to burn fats and sugar for energy:
MITOFORTE: Take four capsules each morning with breakfast.

For CoQ10:

MAG-10: Take one capsule daily with a meal.

For extra B-complex vitamins:

COFACTOR B: Take one capsule daily with food.

For liver detoxification pathways:

N-ACETYL-CYSTEINE (NAC): Take one capsule daily with food. *Take one bottle and then discontinue.*

For additional support:

SUPREME MULTIVITAMIN (WITHOUT IRON): Take four capsules daily with a meal.

For general nutritional support:

Consider intravenous nutritional therapy as done before, as needed.

* * *

While going through the program, all the patient's symptoms resolved, including her depression. She was successfully weaned off her Paxil. In summary, Dr. Neustadt's treatment plan developed specifically for this patient demonstrates several key points. First, every treatment plan with this integrative medical approach is customized to the patient's needs. No two treatment plans are the same. In conventional medicine, physicians talk about customizing treatment plans, but limited time allocation, restricted knowledge of the spectrum of possibilities of causality, and an inability to understand and use these functional biochemical tests precludes physicians from even approaching the problem in an integrative, holistic way.

Second, although this plan may appear quite complicated and overwhelming to the reader, and indeed to the patient, compliance with this approach is greater than 95%. Why? One reason is that by the time most people elect to try this approach to their health they've been sick for many years without any relief. In fact their condition is usually getting worse. They are highly motivated to try a scientifically rigorous alternative.

Third, another crucial factor to the high compliance rate is because people experience improvement exceedingly fast, usually within seventy-two hours. They have finally found hope in a way that empowers them to help heal themselves. The conventional medical system removes patients' sense of power to help themselves and creates a socialized helplessness. In contrast, this functional medical approach allows patients to participate in their own health care with their clinician, whom they expect will help them to achieve concrete results. The true results patients seek are those results that are not merely eliminating symptoms, as severe as they may be, but are instead attacking the root causes and curing them.

Chapter Five

Irritable Bowel Syndrome

Irritable Bowel Syndrome (IBS), as the name implies, is a group of symptoms that include gas and bloating, abdominal discomfort, and constipation or diarrhea. IBS is a diagnosis of exclusion. It is diagnosed after other conditions, such as irritable bowel disease (IBD), have been ruled out.

IBS affects 10-20% of the population at any given time[87-89] with women being affected three times more frequently than men.[90] More than 2.2 million prescriptions are written annually for this condition.[91] Tragically, women with IBS are three times more likely to receive a hysterectomy[92] and report more surgical procedures, such as appendectomies.[93]

The total annual costs (direct and indirect) of treating IBS in the United States have been estimated to be approximately $30 billion, excluding prescription and over-the-counter drug costs.[94] Up to 75% of the economic burden is from reduced workforce activity.[87] Patients with IBS miss about three times as many days from work or school annually as people without this condition.[88] Up to 3.5 million physicians' visits each year are because of IBS symptoms.[95, 96] Patients with IBS cost employers 50% more than employees without IBS. The total average cost to employers per employee with IBS was $6,364 compared to $4,245 for employees without IBS. The difference in cost is due to outpatient, office and prescription drug care and medically related work absenteeism costs. Employers spend $1,060 per employee per year on prescription drugs for IBS.

With the biochemical testing approach, a large percentage of these costs and procedures, and the emotional and physical suffering that goes along with them, would be completely unnecessary.

Dr. Pieczenik

For IBS, conventional medicine likes to treat the multiplicity of symptoms and does not understand the underlying causes. The irony is that although no specific motility or structural abnormalities have been consistently demonstrated, the conventional medical community continues to prescribe medications that primarily affect GI motility. Antispamodic medications of the anticholinergic class, such as dicyclomine (Benyl), hyoscyamine sulfate (Levsin); synthetic opiods such as diphenoxylate hydrochloride (Lomotil), loperamide (Imodium). Antidepressants are also considered part of the treatment, including imipramine (Tofranil), amitryptyline (Elavil, actually an anticholinergic), and more.

Conventional medicine, just like functional medicine, looks at two basic factors: the motility of the gut and the psychological predeterminants of this condition (e.g., stress). However, conventional medicine merely tries to attenuate these symptoms instead of identifying and removing the underlying causes. Yes, psychological counseling may be prescribed, but unless the cause of the physical pain is identified and removed, you can only go so far with the psychological determinants.

Dr. Neustadt

There are many natural treatments for IBS that can help. In a 2001 study published in the journal *Behaviour Research and Therapy*, meditating 30 minutes a day for six weeks significantly decreased diarrhea, bloating, flatulence and belching in one study.[97] Additionally, 23% of the participants had decreased headaches, 23% had decreased backache, 8% had less TMJ discomfort, 8% had a decrease in their high blood pressure, 8% noted improvements in their sleep and 31% had less "jumpiness." Many also reported increased enjoyment in life (46%), energy (39%), and concentration (31%), while also reporting less worry (31%), depression (31%) and anxiety (39%). For those who practiced meditation, 86% experienced improved symptoms. Not surprisingly, there were no side effects.

Dietary allergies can contribute to IBS symptoms and eliminating them can lead to dramatic improvement. A systematic review of the role dietary allergies play in IBS, published in 2006 in the journal *Neurogastroenterology and Motility*, concluded that eliminating dietary allergens can lead to an improvement in up to 71% of IBS sufferers.[98] Blood tests for IgG antibodies and the allergy elimination-challenge protocol are most sensitive at detecting food intolerances that contribut to IBS. In an elimination-challenge protocol, patients follow a hypoallergenic diet for a prescribed period of time and track their symptoms in a journal. Then they methodically, and with guidance from a clinician, reintroduce foods one at a time. If symptoms return with specific foods, those are eliminated from their diet altogether, perhaps not forever, but for a while.

While the allergy elimination-challenge protocol is the gold standard for detecting food allergies, the vast majority of patients cannot complete the protocol. Instead, they may make the mistake of challenging themselves with something that is not a pure representative of a food. For example, when challenging wheat, a person has to eat pure wheat; not a piece of bread, which contains other ingredients. Additionally, the elimination-challenge protocol can take months to complete, and is so restrictive that most people cannot follow it for that long.

The more clinically relevant approach is the IgG food allergy test. For children Dr. Neustadt will order an IgG 30-food allergy panel. In this panel the sample is obtained via a fingerstick, thereby avoiding the trauma to the child of a full venous blood draw. For adults, a serum IgG 90-food allergy panel is ordered. These tests, while not conventionally ordered, are more relevant to IBS and other delayed-type hypersensitivity reactions than an IgE blood test. However, an IgE test can be negative when an IgG test is positive.

Dietary supplements, including probiotics and peppermint can also benefit people with IBS. Probiotics, which are beneficial gut bacteria, have been the subject of multiple clinical trials of IBS. In one study, volunteers received 1×10^{10} cfu (colony forming units) of *Lactobacillus salivarius* or *Bifidobacterium infantis* in a malted drink or placebo once daily. Those who took the *Bifidobacterium infantis* probiotic experienced a significant improvement in abdominal pain, bloating and bowel movement difficulty or urgency.[99] A second study showed that symptoms decreased in 76% of volunteers who took a probiotic drink containing *Lactobacillus rhamnosus* GG, *Lactobacillus rhamnosus* LC705, *Bifidobacterium breve* Bb999 and *Propionibacterium freudenreichii* delivering $8\text{-}9 \times 10^9$ cfu daily for six months.[100] Clinical improvement noted in this study was likely due to a pre-existing dysbiosis, which was corrected using probiotics.

Enteric-coated peppermint oil has also been shown in a clinical trial to decrease pain in children with IBS.[101] In this clinical trial, 42 children received enteric coated peppermint oil capsules for 2 weeks, at which time 71% of the volunteers in the peppermint oil group reported improvement in symptoms compared with 43% in the placebo group.

Case: IBS in a Forty-nine-year-old Woman

A forty-nine-year-old woman complained of diarrhea multiple times a week with past diagnoses of diarrhea-predominant IBS and depression. She would experience bouts of urgency several times a day, during which she would be forced to stop anything she was doing to rush to the bathroom where she would have diarrhea. She also was taking 40 mg of Prozac for the depression. Her health goal was to test for the possible underlying causes of her IBS so that she could get rid of it once and for all.

Her MetaCT 400 test results revealed severe allergies to dairy; functional hypothyroidism (low T3); deficiencies in all ten essential amino acids and some non-essential amino acids; multiple essential mineral deficiencies (magnesium, zinc, and manganese); elevated free radical damage to lipids and DNA, which are risk factors for heart disease and cancer; mercury toxicity, a risk factor for depression and irritability; vitamin D insufficiency, a risk factor for colorectal cancer, osteoporosis, and cervical cancer; decreased ability to burn fats and carbohydrates for energy production; borderline vitamin B12 deficiency, a risk factor for dementia; intestinal bacterial dysbiosis, a risk factor for malabsorption and nutritional deficiencies; and iron deficiency (low ferritin). Her test results, below, explained her IBS and depression.

Her MetaCT 400 test results showed:

Food allergies			
Egg, White	1,036	Severe	+5
Egg, Yolk	661	Mod	+4
Intestinal Bacterial Infections			
Bacillus sp.		2.9E+008	H
Citrobacter sp.		1.9E+009	H
Pseudomonas sp.		2.0E+008	H
Salmonella sp.		4.3E+008	H

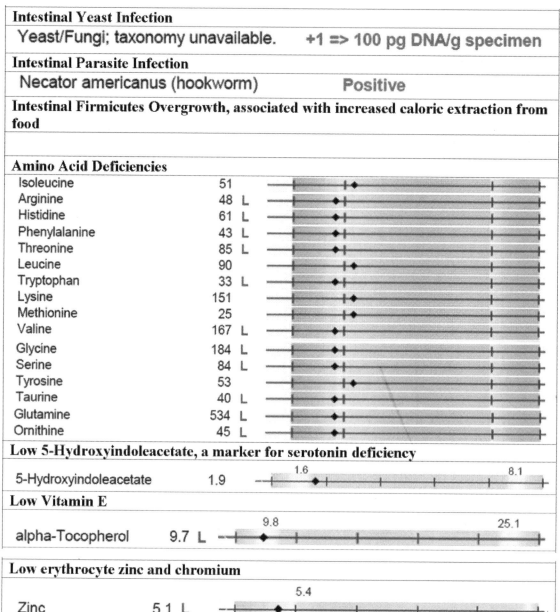

Intestinal Yeast Infection

Yeast/Fungi; taxonomy unavailable.   +1 => 100 pg DNA/g specimen

Intestinal Parasite Infection

Necator americanus (hookworm)   Positive

Intestinal Firmicutes Overgrowth, associated with increased caloric extraction from food

Amino Acid Deficiencies

Isoleucine	51	
Arginine	48	L
Histidine	61	L
Phenylalanine	43	L
Threonine	85	L
Leucine	90	
Tryptophan	33	L
Lysine	151	
Methionine	25	
Valine	167	L
Glycine	184	L
Serine	84	L
Tyrosine	53	
Taurine	40	L
Glutamine	534	L
Ornithine	45	L

Low 5-Hydroxyindoleacetate, a marker for serotonin deficiency

| 5-Hydroxyindoleacetate | 1.9 | | 1.6 | | 8.1 |

Low Vitamin E

| alpha-Tocopherol | 9.7 L | | 9.8 | | 25.1 |

Low erythrocyte zinc and chromium

| Zinc | 5.1 L | | 5.4 |
| Chromium | 2.5 L | | 3.0 |

This woman was placed on a therapeutic elimination diet, her bacterial infection was treated, and her nutritional deficiencies were addressed with dietary supplements and dietary modification. After six weeks of being on the program, her diarrhea was decreased by 80%, and she no longer had any urgency. After twelve weeks her IBS was decreased by 90%, and she no longer experienced gas/bloating or diarrhea except when she would eat dairy. Her mood had also improved during this period. She reported feeling "calmer," and she began working with her physician to discontinue her antidepressant medication.

Treatment Plan

Summary of Results:
(1) Major food allergy to dairy; (2) functional hypothyroidism (low T3); (3) deficient in all ten essential amino acids and some non-essential amino acids; (4) multiple essential mineral deficiencies (magnesium, zinc, and manganese); (5) elevated free radical damage to lipids and DNA; (6) mercury toxicity; (7) vitamin D insufficiency; (8) decreased ability to burn fats and carbohydrates for energy production; (9) borderline vitamin B12 deficiency; (10) intestinal bacterial dysbiosis; (11) iron deficiency (low ferritin); (12) altered fatty acid ratio. These abnormalities in your lab results correspond to the following symptoms and disease risk factors: depression, fatigue, insomnia, irritable bowel syndrome, increased dementia risk, increased cancer risk, increased cardiovascular disease risk, and osteoporosis risk. *Note: All laboratory abnormalities may be corrected.*

Diet:
AVOID all *casein (a protein found in high quantities in dairy products), milk, and all dairy products* for eight weeks, and then reintroduce them into your diet.

Lifestyle:
STRESS REDUCTION: Your laboratory reports point to chronic high levels of stress as being a major underlying cause for your symptoms and nutritional insufficiencies. Decrease stress by practicing yoga, going on slow walks, or otherwise identifying ways to relax.

Exercise: Decrease exercise intensity for the next six weeks. When doing a cardio workout, *only* exercise to the point at which you begin to perspire, and then stop. If you do weight-bearing exercise, do not push yourself too hard; exercise only to the point at which you begin to feel a muscle burn and then immediately stop. These recommendations will increase your metabolism and heart rate without putting too much added stress on your body. After six weeks on the plan you may be able to resume a more strenuous exercise regimen.

For intestinal bacterial overgrowth:

BERBERINE FORTE Take one capsule twice daily with food for two months.

ENTEROPRO: Take one capsule daily with food. *Keep refrigerated.*

For low amino acids:

Note: You may combine the powders and take them at the same time.

CUSTOMIZED AMINO ACID BLEND: Use as directed on the bottle for three months.

GLUTAMINE RX: Mix one teaspoon twice daily in water and drink.

For low vitamins and minerals:

SUPREME MULTIVITAMIN (WITHOUT IRON): Take four capsules daily with a meal.

REJUVAMAG: Take two capsules each night before bed.

CALCIUM COMPLEX: Take two capsules daily.

MAG-10: Take one capsule daily with a meal.

PROMINERALS: Take three capsules daily with food. *Take one bottle and then discontinue.*

SUPER D3: Take one capsule daily with food.

MITOFORTE: Take two capsules each morning with breakfast.

B-12 SUBLINGUAL: Dissolve one lozenge under the tongue daily.

COFACTOR B: Take one capsule daily with food.

For elevated free radical damage to lipids and DNA:

PROTECT DM: Take one capsule daily.

CURCUMIN PRO: Take two tablets twice daily.

EMERGEN-C: Take three to six packets daily as tolerated.

Case: IBS in a Thirty-one-year-old Woman

As this case demonstrates, the underlying causes of IBS are not always the same, and therefore this woman's treatment plan is quite different from the previous case. This case is that of a thirty-one-year-old woman who suffered for many years from severe bouts of diarrhea. They were so debilitating that she also suffered from extreme anxiety to the point where she refused to board a plane or even take a vacation with her husband. Not surprisingly, she also suffered from depression, abdominal pain, and social phobia. She had also been trying to get pregnant for ten months without conceiving.

She had originally gone to see Dr. Neustadt a year earlier and decided not to take his recommendations to get tested. However, her symptoms persisted and even got worse. It turned out that a close friend of hers had been evaluated by Dr. Neustadt and her life-long depression and insomnia were cured. The point here is that some people need reassurance from a friend that this functional and holistic approach may help them before they are willing to set aside their skepticism and fear and give it a try. Drs. Pieczenik and Neustadt find this phenomenon very interesting and common, since patients don't question the legitimacy of the allopathic approach even though they don't understand the science behind it either. But in terms of the functional medicine approach, they often need a reference point of credibility in order to allow them to get to the point that they'll follow this approach. This is the same for other approaches besides the functional testing, including prolotherapy and mesotherapy.

Her test results showed:

Moderate and severe food allergies to common foods			
Beef	410	Mod	+3
Casein	872	Mod	+4
Egg, White	1,184	Severe	+5
Egg, Yolk	894	Mod	+4
Lamb	74	Mild	+1
Milk	754	Mod	+4
Vanilla	462	Mod	+3
Almond	164	Mod	+3
Pistachio	153	Mod	+3
Peanut	348	Mod	+3

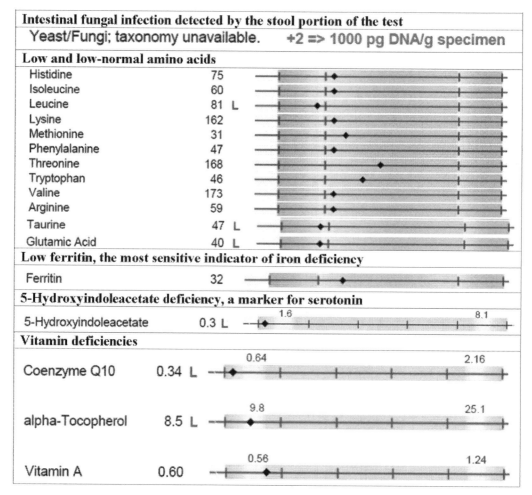

Intestinal fungal infection detected by the stool portion of the test
Yeast/Fungi; taxonomy unavailable.   +2 => 1000 pg DNA/g specimen

Low and low-normal amino acids

Histidine	75
Isoleucine	60
Leucine	81 L
Lysine	162
Methionine	31
Phenylalanine	47
Threonine	168
Tryptophan	46
Valine	173
Arginine	59
Taurine	47 L
Glutamic Acid	40 L

Low ferritin, the most sensitive indicator of iron deficiency

| Ferritin | 32 |

5-Hydroxyindoleacetate deficiency, a marker for serotonin

| 5-Hydroxyindoleacetate | 0.3 L |

Vitamin deficiencies

Coenzyme Q10	0.34 L
alpha-Tocopherol	8.5 L
Vitamin A	0.60

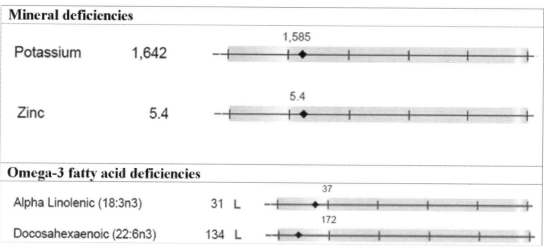

Mineral deficiencies

| Potassium | 1,642 |
| Zinc | 5.4 |

Omega-3 fatty acid deficiencies

| Alpha Linolenic (18:3n3) | 31 L |
| Docosahexaenoic (22:6n3) | 134 L |

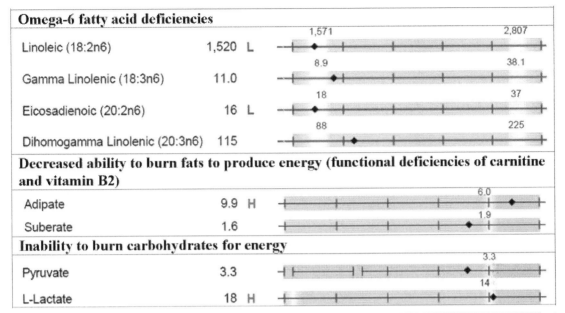

Omega-6 fatty acid deficiencies		
Linoleic (18:2n6)	1,520 L	1,571 ——◆—————————— 2,807
Gamma Linolenic (18:3n6)	11.0	8.9 —◆————————— 38.1
Eicosadienoic (20:2n6)	16 L	18 —◆————————— 37
Dihomogamma Linolenic (20:3n6)	115	88 ———◆———————— 225

Decreased ability to burn fats to produce energy (functional deficiencies of carnitine and vitamin B2)

Adipate	9.9 H	6.0 ————————◆—
Suberate	1.6	1.9 ——————◆——

Inability to burn carbohydrates for energy

Pyruvate	3.3	3.3 ———————◆—
L-Lactate	18 H	14 ————————◆

Deficiencies in Kreb's Cycle intermediates, indicated inefficient ATP production. Note: Malate is a sensitive indicator of CoQ10 deficiency

Citrate	515 H	431 ————————◆—
a-Ketoglutarate	54.7 H	21.0 —————————◆
Malate	2.4 H	1.5 —————————◆—

Biotin deficiency

ß-Hydroxyisovalerate	4.3	4.7 ———————◆—

Impaired liver metabolic pathways

Orotate	0.38	0.44 ———————◆—
Sulfate	118 L	123 —◆——————— 343

Aluminum toxicity

Aluminum	65 H	61 —————————◆—

This woman was placed on customized treatment plan (see below) to treat the underlying causes of her symptoms and rebuild her health. She was told to stop trying to get pregnant until the completion of the three-month treatment plan until repeat toxic metals testing showed she no longer had dangerous levels of toxic metals. After just a few days of complete avoidance of dietary allergens, she reported a complete resolution of her IBS symptoms. She no longer had severe abdominal pain and diarrhea.

At her two-week follow-up appointment, she reported that she continued to improve and felt much better. One important aspect of this plan for her, as it is with many people who are diagnosed with food allergies, is that she began to advocate for herself when she would go out to eat and question the waiters to ensure that she was getting food that wouldn't harm her. This empowerment for her was very important. It is quite common for many people, and women in particular. It is the first time in their lives that they actually act proactively about their health and place themselves first without feeling guilty.

Treatment Plan

Diet:
AVOID all *beef, dairy, dairy-containing products, casein (a protein found in high concentrations in dairy and also used as a food additive), eggs, and all egg-containing products, peanuts, vanilla, almonds, and pistachios* for eight weeks, then reintroduce them into your diet one at a time.

For gut rebuilding:
GLUTAMINE RX: Mix one teaspoon twice daily in water and drink.

For low ferritin (iron deficiency):
FERROSOLVE: Take one capsule twice daily. *Note: Taking with some vitamin C can increase its absorption.*

For CoQ10:
COENZYME Q10 POWDER: Take two scoops dissolved in eight ounces of water daily with a meal.

For vitamin D:
Go in the sun for twenty minutes without sunscreen, and then put sunscreen on. This will stimulate vitamin D production in your body. Sunscreen blocks vitamin D production.

For potassium:
K+2 POTASSIUM: Take one capsule daily with food. Take one bottle and then discontinue.

For zinc:

AN-30: Take one capsule twice daily with a meal. Take one bottle and then discontinue.

For additional vitamins and minerals:

SUPREME FEM MULTIVITAMIN (WITH IRON): Take four capsules daily with a meal.

For fatty acids:

CARLSON'S COD LIVER OIL: Take one tablespoon (equivalent of 3 teaspoons) daily. Keep refrigerated.

For ability to burn fats and sugars for energy:

MITOFORTE: Take four capsules each morning with breakfast.

For biotin:

BIOTIN 5000 MCG: Take one capsule daily.

For liver detoxification pathways:

N-ACETYL-CYSTEINE (NAC): Take one capsule daily. Take one bottle and then discontinue.

For toxic metals (aluminum):

CALCIUM-DISODIUM-EDTA INTRAVENOUS THERAPY to chelate toxic metals. Expect a minimum of ten treatments, spaced one week apart. Whole blood toxic metals will be retested after ten treatments.

Chapter Six

Irritable Bowel Disease

Irritable bowel disease (IBD) is a group of two diseases that includes Crohn's disease (CD) and ulcerative colitis (UC). UC usually affects only the innermost lining of the large intestine (colon) and rectum. It occurs only through continuous stretches of the colon, unlike Crohn's disease, which occurs in patches anywhere in the digestive tract and often spreads deep into the layers of affected tissues. CD is also known as "regional enteritis." CD can affect any part of the gastrointestinal tract from mouth to anus, whereas UC primarily affects the descending colon.

UC is a chronic, recurring disease of the large bowel. When UC affects the colon, inflammation and ulcers, or sores, form in the lining of the colon. The disease may involve the entire colon (pancolitis), only the rectum (ulcerative proctitis), or more commonly, somewhere between the two.

The causes of CD and UC are unknown. Some experts believe there may be a defect in the immune system in which the body's antibodies actually injure the colon. Others speculate that an unidentified microorganism or germ is responsible for the disease. It is probable that a combination of factors, including heredity, may be involved in the cause.

These disorders typically begin gradually, with crampy abdominal pain and diarrhea that is sometimes bloody. In more severe cases, diarrhea is very severe and frequent. Loss of appetite and weight loss occur. The patient may become weak and very sick. When the UC is localized to the rectum, the symptoms are rectal urgency and passage of small amounts of bloody stool. Usually symptoms tend to come and go, and there may be long periods without any symptoms at all.

Diagnosis of Crohn's disease and UC can be suspected from the symptoms. Certain blood and stool tests are performed to rule out an infection that can mimic the disorder. Sigmoidoscopy or colonoscopy typically reveals a characteristic pattern of lesions in the bowels. A barium enema x-ray of the colon may be needed at some point during the course of the disease.

Diet and Emotions

There are no foods known to injure the bowel. However, during an acute phase of the disease, bulky foods, milk, and milk products can increase diarrhea and cramping. Generally, the patient is advised to eat a healthy, well-balanced diet with adequate protein and calories. A multiple vitamin is often recommended. Iron may be prescribed if anemia is present.

Stress and anxiety may aggravate symptoms of the disorder, but are not believed to cause it or make it worse. Any chronic disease can produce a serious emotional reaction in the patient. This can usually be handled through discussion with the physician. There are excellent support groups available in most communities.

Surgery

For patients with longstanding disease that is difficult or impossible to control with medicine, surgery is a welcomed option. In these rare cases, the patient's lifestyle and general health have been significantly affected. Surgical removal of the colon cures the disease and returns good health and a normal lifestyle to the patient. In the past a permanent bag, or ileostomy, was required for this surgery. Advances in surgery now can avoid this problem. The colon is removed and a pouch or reservoir is created from the small intestine. Three to six liquid bowel movements occur daily. Most patients are extremely pleased with this new surgery.

No one is quite sure what triggers inflammation in Crohn's disease and UC. The conventional treatment for Crohn's disease and UC are nearly identical. Most patients with these diseases respond well to treatment and go about their lives with few interruptions. However, some attacks may be quite severe, requiring a period of bowel rest, hospitalization, and intravenous treatment. In rare cases, emergency surgery is required. The disease can affect nutrition, causing poor growth during childhood and adolescence. Liver, skin, eye, or joint (arthritis) problems occasionally occur, even before the bowel symptoms develop. Other problems can include narrowing and partial blocking of the bile ducts, which carry bile from the liver to the intestine. Fortunately, there is much that can be done about all of these complications.

In long-standing ulcerative colitis, the major concern is colon cancer. The risk of developing colon cancer increases significantly when the disorder begins in childhood, has been present for eight to ten years, or when there is a family history of colon cancer. In these situations, it is particularly important to perform regular and thorough surveillance of the colon, even when there are no symptoms. Analysis of colon biopsies performed during colonoscopy can often predict if colon cancer will occur. In these cases, preventive surgery is recommended.

There are several types of medical treatments available for CD and UC. Prednisone provides highly effective results at decreasing inflammation. A high dose is often used initially to bring the disorder under control. However, it is not without risk. Since a major risk of prednisone therapy is osteoporosis, the authors recommend that any patients on prednisone consider treatments that can decrease the risk of this dangerous side effect. The only natural treatment shown to do this is high doses of vitamin K_2 as MK4.

MK4 exerts a powerful influence on bone building, especially in osteoporosis, and in Japan has been accepted as an osteoporosis treatment.[102] It is a fat-soluble vitamin that is a coenzyme for a vitamin K-dependent carboxylase enzyme that catalyzes carboxylation of the amino acid glutamic acid, resulting in its conversion to gamma-carboxyglutamic acid (Gla). This carboxylation reaction is essential for formation of bone collagen, which allows bone to deform upon impact, for example during a fall, without fracturing. Although vitamin K-dependent gamma-carboxylation occurs only on specific glutamic acid residues in a small number of proteins, it is critical to the calcium-binding function of those proteins.

Three vitamin K-dependent proteins have been isolated in bone—osteocalcin, matrix Gla protein (MGP), and protein S. Osteocalcin is a protein that is synthesized by osteoblasts. The synthesis of osteocalcin by osteoblasts is regulated by the active form of vitamin D, $1,25\text{-}(OH)_2D_3$, or calcitriol. The mineral-binding capacity of osteocalcin requires vitamin K-dependent gamma-carboxylation of three glutamic acid residues. Matrix Gla protein (MGP), has been found in bone, cartilage, and soft tissue, including blood vessels. Results of animal studies suggest that MGP prevents the calcification of soft tissue and cartilage while facilitating normal bone growth and development. Multiple randomized, double-blind, placebo-controlled clinical trials have shown significant decreases in undercarboxylated osteocalcin (ucOC) in volunteers supplemented with 45 mg of MK4 with and without the addition of calcium and vitamin D_3 compared to controls.[103-106]

It's important to note that vitamin K_1 (phylloquinone) is preferentially used by the liver as a clotting factor. MK4, on the other hand, is used preferentially in other organs, such as the brain, vasculature, breasts, and kidneys. Coagulation studies in humans using 45 mg per day of as MK4[105] and even up to 135 mg/day (45 mg tid) of MK4[107] showed no significant increase in pathologic coagulation risk. Even doses in rats as high as 250 mg/kg body weight did not alter the tendency for blood-clot formation to occur.[108]

A 2006 meta-analysis published in the *Archives of Internal Medicine* by Sarah Cockayne, MSc, Joy Adams, PhD, Susan Lanham-New, PhD, and colleagues, at the University of York in England, evaluated clinical trials on vitamin K_2 and fracture risk.[109] They identified thirteen randomized, controlled trials of the effect of vitamin K_2 on osteoporosis. Of those, seven had fracture risk as an end point and so were included in their meta-analysis. They concluded that 45 mg of MK4 may decrease vertebral fracture by 60%, hip fracture by 73%, and all nonvertebral fractures by 81%.

An excellent review of vitamin K_2 by Stephen Plaza, ND, and Davis Lamson, ND, was published in 2005 in the journal *Alternative Medicine Review.*[110] In this article they reviewed clinical trials using MK4 that showed increases in BMD and/or reduction in fracture risk in volunteers who had bone loss from anorexia nervosa, Parkinson's disease, biliary cirrhosis, and stroke and in volunteers who were taking prednisone and leuprolide; in other volunteers, it increased the efficacy of bisphosphonate medications.

It's important for clinicians to understand that there are primarily two forms of vitamin K_2 that are commercially available. These are MK4 and MK7. MK4 is a synthetic form of vitamin K_2 and the agent used in the clinical trials mentioned above. MK7 is produced by bacterial fermentation of soy, appears to have a longer half life then MK4, and can also decrease serum uOC.[111] However, only MK4 has demonstrated the ability to decrease fracture risk, the clinically relevant end point, in randomized, controlled clinical trials. Based on this research, the authors' created the only dietary supplement that contains the dose (45 mg) and form of MK4 used in the clinical trials. This formula is called Osteo-K and is being prescribed all over the country by clinicians for their patients.

Other anti-inflammatory drugs are also available to treat the symptoms of UC. They are sulfasalazine (Azulfidine), olsalazine (Dipentum), mesalamine (Asacol, Pentasa and Rowasa), and balsalazide (Colazal).

Medications such as azathioprine (Imuran), 6-MP (Purinethol), cyclosporine (Neoral, Sandimmune), and methotrexate (Rheumatrex) suppress the immune system and at times are effective as well.

Dr. Pieczenik

Dr. Pieczenik's father, a medical doctor himself, worked with Dr. Crohn, who was Dr. Pieczenik's family physician. Dr. Crohn's ability to diagnose was impressive, given the period when medicine didn't have advanced technologies and procedures such as colonoscopy. However, the barium enema did exist at that time. This radiological procedure, which utilized a high-dose of X-rays in combination with taking barium to enhance the contrast on the X-ray, allowed clinicians to see the outlines of ulcers within the bowels. This was not a very precise technique, and so false negatives were very high. It could be said that the treatment was always the same—decrease stress, high doses of steroids, and high doses of salicylates. The distinct caveat was that symptoms would flare up again under acute stress or spontaneously. Unexplicable remissions may occur from time to time, but the prognosis was one of a chronic, deteriorating disease. The only other intervention, which is still used today, is surgical resection of the bowel. This was in the 1950s. Almost nothing's changed the subsequent sixty years of so-called "medical progress."

Dr. Neustadt

The subsequent testing and treatment approach describes the functional biochemical paradigm for helping patients with these conditions.

Case: Crohn's Disease in a Sixty-five-year-old Woman

A sixty-five-year-old woman presented to Montana Integrative Medicine with CD. She had been diagnosed forty-three years earlier in 1964 and had undergone a hemicolectomy. She suffered from extreme fatigue, insomnia, weakness, and chronic post-nasal drip.

Her test results revealed deficiencies in branched chain amino acids (leucine, isoleucine, and valine) required to form muscle; low minerals (magnesium, copper, and vanadium); extremely low vitamin D2; elevated free radical damage to DNA, a risk factor for cancer; an intestinal fungal infection; and decreased ability to utilize sugars to produce energy due to functional deficiencies in B-complex vitamins and lipoic acid. Additionally, she had food allergies to milk, casein (a protein found in high concentrations in milk and dairy products, and added to many packaged foods), eggs, garlic, and mustard greens.

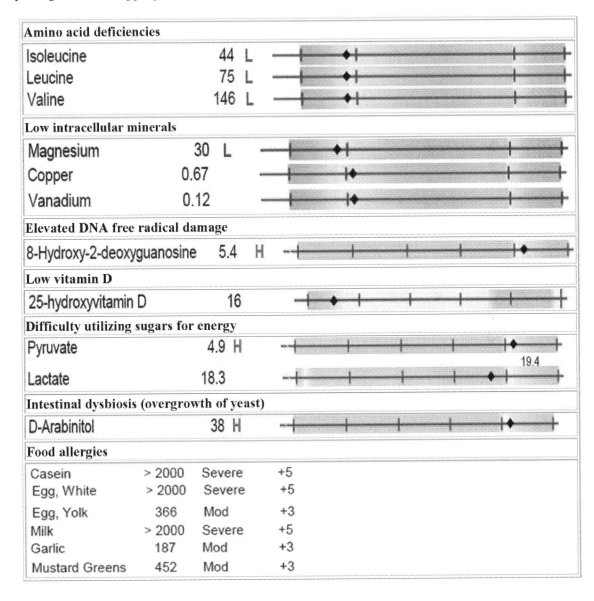

Amino acid deficiencies			
Isoleucine	44	L	
Leucine	75	L	
Valine	146	L	

Low intracellular minerals			
Magnesium	30	L	
Copper	0.67		
Vanadium	0.12		

Elevated DNA free radical damage			
8-Hydroxy-2-deoxyguanosine	5.4	H	

Low vitamin D		
25-hydroxyvitamin D	16	

Difficulty utilizing sugars for energy			
Pyruvate	4.9	H	
Lactate	18.3		19.4

Intestinal dysbiosis (overgrowth of yeast)		
D-Arabinitol	38	H

Food allergies			
Casein	> 2000	Severe	+5
Egg, White	> 2000	Severe	+5
Egg, Yolk	366	Mod	+3
Milk	> 2000	Severe	+5
Garlic	187	Mod	+3
Mustard Greens	452	Mod	+3

She was placed on a customized program that included dietary recommendations, targeted nutrient therapies to provide highly-concentrated sources of nutrients, and a protocol to eliminate the infection in her intestines. After three months on the program, she reported that her energy had doubled and that, "I haven't felt this good in twenty-five years." Her post-nasal drip had cleared up, she was sleeping better, and she felt stronger and more positive about herself and her health.

Treatment Plan

Diet:

AVOID all *casein, dairy, dairy products, eggs, garlic, and mustard greens* for eight weeks, then reintroduce them into your diet. See the handout on alternatives to milk products.

For intestinal fungal overgrowth:

NYSTATIN TABLETS, 500,000 units twice daily for three months.

ENTEROPRO: Take one capsule daily with food.

For amino acids:

BCAA POWDER: Take one scoop per day in a liquid of your choosing. Take one bottle and then discontinue.

GLUTAMINE RX: Mix one teaspoon twice daily in water and drink.

For low vitamin D:

SUPER D3: Take one capsule daily with food.

For vitamins and minerals:

SUPREME MULTIVITAMIN (WITHOUT IRON) Take four capsules daily with a meal.

Case: Ulcerative Colitis in a Fifty-five-year-old Woman

A fifty-five-year-old woman suffered a single attack of ulcerative colitis in January 2008. A colonoscopy revealed lesions in her descending colon, and she was placed on a round of prednisone by her gastroenterologist. Dr. Neustadt ordered a stool test for her that revealed an infection of *Trichuris* sp., commonly called whipworm. Her microbial stool analysis revealed:

Parasitic Protozoans

Trichuris sp.   Positive   Neg

She was also tested for and shown to be deficient in iron and vitamin D. She was placed on the following treatment plan.

Treatment Plan

For the roundworm:
Rx Mebendazole 100 mg orally twice daily for three days.

After your finish the three days of Mebendazole, then start:
PARA-GARD: Take one capsule three times daily for two days, then two capsules three times daily for two days, then three capsules three times daily thereafter. Take all capsules between meals, if possible.

ACTIVATED CHARCOAL: Take two capsules after eating lunch and two capsules two hours later; repeat with and after dinner.

FERROSOLVE: Take one capsule daily with or without food.

VITAMIN D3: Take one capsule daily with food.

* * *

It's important to note here that Drs. Neustadt and Pieczenik do not necessarily believe that this infection caused her UC. However, after completing the treatment plan, the patient returned to her gastroenterologist, who performed another colonoscopy. The patient reported that her gastroenterologist told her that he had never seen anyone heal so quickly from the lesions that he had previously detected.

Whether the patient was cured or not from this approach is not known. However, she clearly had marked and quick improvement. What's noteworthy here is that the testing method for analyzing the stool is much more sensitive and specific that the traditional O&Px3, as the authors discussed earlier in the book. The new testing technology may end up revolutionizing the treatment for UC, and possibly, Crohn's disease, but requires more study. What's important in this case is that the approach included two factors that are commonly overlooked in conventional, symptom-oriented medicine: (1) remove any detected infection; and (2) build the immune system to allow it to heal more quickly.

Chapter Seven

Gastroesophageal Reflux Disorder (GERD)

As previously discussed in the section, "Heal the Gut, Heal the Body," GERD may be caused by too little stomach acid, infections, and food allergies. Symptoms of GERD include substernal burning as the stomach acid refluxes into the esophagus; hoarse throat; difficulty swallowing (dysphagia); a dry, hacking cough; chest pain; breathing difficulties, particularly at night when lying in bed; and mature-onset asthma. GERD may also be caused by a hiatal hernia, which may be improved with surgery, breathing exercises, or manual reduction of the hernia, a technique called "visceral manipulation."

Case: GERD

The following are the actual chart notes, with the patient's identifying information redacted, for this case.

The patient comes in today for evaluation for a myriad of complaints, all of which I've already discussed with her. We will not be able to address all of them in one appointment. She lists as her complaints: head injury, acid reflux, menopause, cholesterol, recurrent infections, depression, and allergies. Patient reports atypical GERD symptoms. She was diagnosed with atypical acid reflux and is not experiencing any burning in her esophagus. Instead, she merely experiences difficulty swallowing.

SOCIAL AND FAMILY HISTORY: Her father died in December 2005, and her mother disinherited her. Since then she has had high levels of stress. Additionally, her daughter had a baby out of wedlock in July 2005. The baby's father is still with the mother; however, they are not married. All three of them are living in a separate apartment, connected to the patient's house.

PAST MEDICAL HISTORY: The patient has a history for traumatic brain injury which she suffered "years ago" in a car accident.

EXERCISE: For stress release, she does stretching exercises daily, which she called the Egoscue method, which she follows up with walking.

SLEEP: She sleeps seven to seven and a half hours per day. She has no sleep phase advance or sleep phase delay. She wakes unrefreshed.

ENERGY: Energy is three out of ten (ten being best). It was higher before last summer.

STRESS: She recently started an art school, which adds additional stress.

DIET RECALL: *Breakfast*: Raw almonds, polenta bread, four to five ounces roast beef, two glasses of water, one quarter cup of milk. *Lunch*: Shrimp poor boy sandwich. *Dinner*: Rice, chicken, artichoke hearts, sun-dried tomatoes, portabella mushrooms, water. *Snacks*: fruit. She drinks no coffee, but she does drink herbal tea. She drinks four to five glasses of water a day.

REVIEW OF SYSTEMS:

She gets headaches frequently, one time per week which are secondary to tight cervical muscles. The headaches are located in the occipital area, and she credits the headaches to be secondary to the car accident. She had three vertebrae (C4–C6) fused as a result of the car accident. She reports weight gain of ten to fifteen in the last year. No tinnitus. No vision changes. She does report allergic rhinitis, which she deemed a "stress allergy." For that she uses Loratidine or Claritin. Positive taste changes. Positive dysphagia, secondary to the acid reflux. Positive chest pressure when tired. She occasionally experiences shortness of breath. She has gas and bloating. Bowel movements: one to two a day. Urine: reports occasional increased frequency of urine, needing to urinate every twenty minutes. She also reports an unpleasant odor currently, and a yellow-green color to the urine. Wound healing: takes more time to heal wounds now than it used to, and she reports getting sick a lot with urinary tract infections. She frequently feels cold, and she occasionally has upper extremity and lower extremity numbness. She occasionally loses her balance. She falls every other day when she is outside a lot. She has never broken any bones secondary to falling. She is experiencing hot flashes daily.

OBJECTIVE: Wt: 123lbs. Ht: 5'3" Temp: 97.8°F BP: 106/66 Pulse: 64 bpm. *Deep Tendon Reflexes*: Achilles: +1 bilaterally with delayed relaxation phase bilaterally. Patellar reflex: +2 bilaterally. *Thyroid:* The isthmus is enlarged. Otherwise no nodules, not tender to palpation.

ASSESSMENT: Traumatic brain injury. Hypercholesterolemia. Depression. GERD.

PLAN: Ordered recent labs, CBC, Met-C, TSH. Recommended she eat three small meals daily with two smaller snacks. I instructed the patient on the composition of complex carbohydrates, protein, and fruits and vegetables that should be on her plate at each meal. I instructed the patient on exercising for thirty minutes per day, five days per week. I put the patient on an elimination diet as an empiric trial for the GERD, having her eliminate chocolate, coffee, tomatoes, citrus foods, and fried foods, and reduce or eliminate sugar and breads from the diet to see if her symptoms of GERD decrease. For other treatment plan recommendations, please see treatment plan printout in her chart.

On a subsequent appointment, this is what was charted:

The patient returns for a follow-up on her symptoms from the GERD and to receive a treatment plan based on the lab results from her amino acid analysis.

She is experiencing hot flashes. She purchased Remifemin on 2/29/06, and she has had no hot flashes since then. She is experiencing no headaches currently, and she has had only two headaches since 2/28/06. She has fallen two to three times since her last appointment on 2/28/06. Her GERD symptoms have essentially been unchanged since starting the elimination diet. Today, she is reporting her throat is slightly sore. She ate spaghetti sauce one time, and it aggravated the symptoms. Also aggravating the symptoms was hot and sour soup from a Chinese food restaurant. She is experiencing longer periods without symptoms; however, she is still experiencing GERD symptoms. She has been strict about eliminating the foods on the list I gave her.

EXERCISE: She is walking up to three quarters of a mile per day

ENERGY: Energy today is four or five out of ten (ten being the best).

OBJECTIVE: The patient is alert and oriented times three and in no acute distress. She ambulated without assistance, and there were no abnormalities in her gait.

ASSESSMENT: Traumatic brain injury. Hypercholesterolemia. Depression. GERD.

PLAN: Branch chain amino acids. Emergen-C. I will order her customized amino-acid supplement for her, which will be shipped directly to her house, and I'm also adding Betaine HCL to her treatment for the GERD to rule out hypochlorhydria.

And subsequent to this appointment, the notes in her chart are:

SUBJECTIVE: The patient comes in today for a follow-up on the treatment plan, to monitor any changes, and to make any adjustments to the treatment plan that may be necessary.

She is currently experiencing depression. She has no suicidal ideations currently and no history of any attempted suicides. She reports that when she feels like taking three baths a day it's part of her depression. She has wanted to take three baths a day for the last week. The depression started one week ago and is better than it was last week. She is not seeing any counselors for the depression, and she is also experiencing decreased appetite with the depression. She is having rashes on her hands. She saw Dr. XYZ for the rash, and he diagnosed her as having a "stress allergy." She is taking all the vitamins that I've prescribed; however, she has only been able to take the amino acid blend and the branch chain amino acid supplements for one and a half weeks, consecutively. When she did, she noticed that many of her symptoms did improve, including the weakness, the fatigue, and the depression.

She is getting a follow-up blood draw next week to test her lipids. I recommended that the patient request a health screen. *She is not having any dysphagia as long as she is taking the Betaine HCL.* She has fallen five times in the last two weeks without injuries.

EXERCISE: She is exercising. She was doing one mile on the treadmill up until last week, when she stopped.

ENERGY: The heat is affecting her and causing increased fatigue.

STRESS: She reports that she has had very high levels of stress recently. She is running an art school and also teaching classes there. Her daughter is now pregnant again and due in July with her second baby. Her daughter, her daughter's boyfriend, and the current baby are still living with her, and they may move out in July. Her high levels of stress worsen her head injury symptoms, which manifest mostly as forgetfulness, increases in hot flashes, and depression. She is now getting hot flashes two to three times per day. When her stress is low, she can go months without any hot flashes. Starting next week she'll have a month off of work, which should help decrease her stress and hopefully ameliorate many of her symptoms.

OBJECTIVE: The patient is alert and oriented times three and in not acute distress. Her affect was noticeably flatter than it had been in the past, and she appeared slightly listless. She was, however, engaged in the conversation and smiled a few times. She ambulated without assistance, and her gait was essentially normal.

ASSESSMENT: 530.81, Esophageal reflux/GERD, 272.0 Pure hypercholesterolemia

PLAN: Stress Reduction. I provided instructions on breathing exercises the patient can do to reduce her stress. I also recommended the patient continue to take her amino acid supplement and all other dietary supplements every day consistently. After she has taken them for three months we can re-evaluate with a blood draw to test her amino acids. I also requested the patient send me copies of the labs that she gets drawn next week. I referred her to a social worker for counseling.

Chapter Eight

Age-Related Degeneration (ARD): Pieczenik-Neustadt Syndrome

Age-related degeneration (ARD) is a term created by Drs. Pieczenik and Neustadt to describe a constellation of symptoms that tend to appear in the elderly. These symptoms may include weakness, fatigue, depression, insomnia, abdominal gas and bloating, diarrhea, brain fog (difficulty processing information), and recurrent infections, such as urinary tract infections (UTI) and/or upper respiratory infections (URI). In these people, conventional medical testing usually does not show any abnormalities, and all treatments merely suppress symptoms.

It is well documented that as we age our risk for nutritional deficiencies increases, and the underlying causes for these symptoms include deficiencies in amino acid, vitamins, minerals and fatty acids, food allergies, and intestinal dysbiosis (overgrowth of bacteria and/or yeast). Biochemical testing can provide the information needed to create a Targeted Nutritional Program™ that can help restore health.

Subclinical nutritional deficiencies can cause muscle catabolism. This pathologic loss of lean body mass is called *sarcopenia*. Both patients in this chapter with ARD suffered from sarcopenia, as well as other diseases. The term sarcopenia was first coined in 1989 by Irwin H. Rosenberg, MD, currently professor of physiology, Friedman School of Nutrition Science & Policy at Tufts University Sackler School of Graduate Biomedical Sciences, who used this term to describe the decrease in lean-body mass that occurs with age. In defining sarcopenia he wrote, "Think of the implication of this decrease in lean-body mass in respect to the physical behavior of elderly subjects. There may be no single feature of age-related decline that could more dramatically affect ambulation, mobility, calorie intake, and overall nutrient intake and status, independence, breathing, etc."[112]

By age 70, voluntary-muscle contractile strength decreases by 20% to 40% in both men and women.[113] Skeletal muscle is the largest reservoir for proteins, containing more than 50% of the body's total protein supply.[114] Loss of muscle mass is a complex process with multiple potential causes, including poor dietary intake, inactivity, neuroendocrine dysregulation, and immune dysfunction, which in turn have been linked to multiple morbid outcomes, including falls, functional decline, osteoporosis, impaired thermoregulation, and glucose intolerance.[115, 116]

The optimal way to increase muscle mass in the elderly is through a multifaceted approach that involves strength training, targeted nutritional therapies such as a high-quality protein powder enriched with branched chain amino acids, a good multiple vitamin and mineral formula, and ensuring adequate caloric intake.

Studies have evaluated with great success the ability to improve muscle mass through exercise and amino acid therapies. In a randomized, open-label, crossover study of 41 elderly (66-84 years) volunteers with sarcopenia, an oral amino acid mixture or an isocaloric placebo was ingested twice daily for 4 months, followed by a 4-month crossover-study period, and concluded with another 8 months of all participants taking the amino-acid mixture.[114]

The total amount of supplemental amino acids was 8 g/day, comprising L-leucine, 2.5 g; L-lysine, 1.3 g; L-isoleucine, 1.25 g; L-valine, 1.25 g; L-threonine, 0.7 g; L-cysteine, 0.3 g; L-histidine, 0.3 g; L-phenylalanine, 0.2 g; L-methionine, 0.1 g; L-tyrosine, 0.06 g; and L-tryptophan, 0.04 g. Volunteers were maintained on controlled diets of 2000 ± 290 kcal/day (55% carbohydrates, 30% lipids, 15% proteins). The researchers evaluated body-mass index, arterial blood pressure, fasting blood glucose, fasting serum insulin, insulin-like growth factor 1 (IGF-1), tumor necrosis factor–α (TNF-α), and the IGF-1/TNF- α ratio.

Results indicate that supplementation with this amino-acid mixture resulted in significant decreases in both fasting blood glucose (*P*<.05) and fasting serum insulin (*P*<.001), as well as TNF-α (*P*<.001), and a significant increase in IGF-1 (*P*<.001) after 16 months compared to baseline. Additionally, according to the authors, "A significant increase in whole-body lean mass was found in both groups of subjects with sarcopenia after 8 and 16 months of amino-acid supplements, by the end of the study reaching the normal values found in age-matched, nonsarcopenic, healthy controls."[114]

While important, sarcopenia is just one component of multisystems failure in ARD. If just sarcopenia were treated, it would not result in overall, long-term clinical benefit, since function would not be restored in other organs.

Dr. Pieczenik

The way we would approach these patients in conventional medicine is to see this patient's symptoms as a compilation of distinct and unrelated complaints. Therefore, each symptom would be evaluated by different specialists and subspecialists: a neurologist for muscle weakness, a urologist for urinary tract infections, a gastroenterologist for loose stools, a psychiatrist for depression and lethargy, and an internist for overall patient management.

Each symptom receives a different type of medication. For muscle pain the doctor may prescribe an anti-inflammatory such as Aleve and/or a muscle relaxant such as Flexor. Additionally, the doctor would look at existing medications such as statin drugs that are known to cause rhabdomyolysis and muscle pain and adjust the medication if necessary. The gastroenterologist would do an upper- and lower-endoscopy. The urologist would prescribe antibiotics and might do a cystoscopy. The point here is that the entire medical system is being called in to evaluate multiple symptoms in isolation instead of integrating the different physiological systems into a comprehensive evaluation that determines the underlying causes and commonalities between these symptoms. At best it is a nightmare. At worst the patient and the family suffer irreversible physical, mental and economic damage.

From a cost perspective, you can imagine how much money the health care system pays to have these people evaluated and treated while all the while these patients are getting worse and having to use medical services even more frequently. So as long as doctors are reimbursed for the number of patients they see each day and for treating just symptoms, and not for the ability to cure patients, the medical system will continue to deteriorate. And chronic, debilitating ailments will be the venue for the inevitable collapse of the system.

Dr. Neustadt

The Pieczenik-Neustadt Syndrome is really the manifestation of interrelated causes that results in the breakdown of different body systems and the multiple expressions of several disease entities. In other words, as in all of medicine, the Law of Parsimony should guide clinical decision making. This law states that the simplest explanation is the most correct one.

In contrast, the basic lens through which an integrative clinician practicing holistic medicine should view this case is by asking the simplest question: why is this person sick, and what is keeping him or her from getting better? It is well documented that with age the risk for nutritional deficiencies increases and that nutritional deficiencies can cause muscle wasting, anorexia, depression, weakness, fatigue, muscle cramps, and immune dysfunction. Additionally, it is well documented that food allergies and gastrointestinal infections can cause gas and bloating, abdominal pain, diarrhea, and constipation. The most fundamental and simplest evaluation then that can be done is to test all of these parameters, which Dr. Neustadt did in the following two cases.

Case: Muscle Wasting, Pain, and Diarrhea in a Sixty-nine-year-old Woman

A sixty-nine-year-old woman went to see Dr. Neustadt at his clinic complaining of extreme fatigue, weakness, muscle pain, severe gas and bloating each time she ate, and a five-year history of loose stools. When she walked less than one block, she experienced painful burning in her muscles. At intake she could only walk half a block and ride for one minute on a stationary bicycle. Additionally, she was unable to stand up from a seated position on the floor without assistance. She was losing strength and balance, which put her at a high risk for falling and hip fractures.

She had been evaluated by gastroenterologists, internists, gynecologists, and urologists at major medical centers around the country. None of them found any abnormalities. Biochemical testing revealed deficiencies in seven out of ten amino acids, low vitamins and minerals required for mitochondrial function, an intestinal bacterial infection, and multiple food allergies.

Low amino acids			
Arginine	50	L	63
Histidine	65	L	67
Isoleucine	45	L	47
Leucine	85	L	87
Lysine	152		135
Methionine	16	L	18
Phenylalanine	53		50
Threonine	72	L	90

Tryptophan	43		42
Valine	168		167
Glycine	154	L	186
Serine	56	L	77

Decreased ability to burn fats to produce energy (functional deficiencies of carnitine and vitamin B2)

Adipate	3.0	H	1.8
Suberate	2.9		3.4
Ethylmalonate	8.8	H	5.5

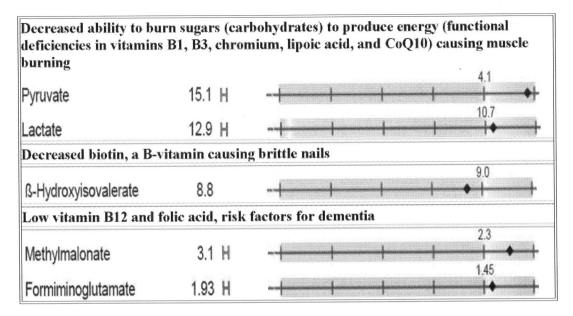

Decreased ability to burn sugars (carbohydrates) to produce energy (functional deficiencies in vitamins B1, B3, chromium, lipoic acid, and CoQ10) causing muscle burning

Pyruvate	15.1 H	4.1
Lactate	12.9 H	10.7

Decreased biotin, a B-vitamin causing brittle nails

ß-Hydroxyisovalerate	8.8	9.0

Low vitamin B12 and folic acid, risk factors for dementia

Methylmalonate	3.1 H	2.3
Formiminoglutamate	1.93 H	1.45

Her treatment consisted of instructions to eliminate all food intolerances, take antibacterial plant extracts for the intestinal infection, high doses of B-complex vitamins with extra vitamin B12, a customized amino acid powder, a high-quality multivitamin and mineral supplement, and physical therapy. Two months later she could walk pain-free for twenty minutes twice daily and ride for ten minutes on an exercise bike. She no longer suffered from diarrhea, and her gas and bloating significantly decreased in frequency and intensity. Additionally, she was able to stand up from a seated position without assistance.

Treatment Plan

The following treatment plan is based on the patient's testing and symptoms. Your test results showed the following: (1) food intolerances to several foods, (2) intestinal dysbiosis (overgrowth of unhealthy bacteria in the intestines), (3) multiple amino acid deficiencies, (4) multiple functional vitamin deficiencies, and (5) vitamin D insufficiency. This treatment plan attempts to correct these dysfunctions.

Diet:
AVOID *all dairy and eggs.* You tested positive for several food intolerances. Read labels carefully—*avoid casein, egg whites, egg yolks, and milk and milk products.*

EXERCISE: Basically, if it feels good, do it. Once burning or pain begins, stop exercising. Do not exercise or do any activities to the point of exhaustion. As amino acids are replensihed, you will likely find yourself feeling stronger and able to do more.

For bacterial dysbiosis:
BERBERINE FORTE: Take one capsule twice daily with food.

ENTEROPRO: Take one capsule daily with food for four months (two bottles).

For amino acids:
CUSTOMIZED AMINO ACID BLEND: Use as directed on the bottle.

BCAA POWDER: Take one scoop per day in a liquid of your choosing.

For cellular energy production:
MITOFORTE: Take four capsules each morning with breakfast.

For B-vitamin deficiencies:
COFACTOR B: Take one capsule daily with food.

SUPREME MULTIVITAMIN (WITHOUT IRON): Take four capsules daily with a meal.

BIOTIN-8: Take one capsule daily.

B-12 SUBLINGUAL: Dissolve one lozenge under the tongue daily.

FA-8 FOLIC ACID: Take one capsule daily.

For vitamin D insufficiency:
SUPER D3: Take one capsule daily with food.

For inflammation:
CURCUMIN PRO: Take one tablet twice daily.

VITAL MIXED ASCORBATES: Mix one scoop twice daily in water, and take with meals.

Case: Weight Loss, Weakness, Gas and Bloating in an Eight-one-year-old Man

An eighty-one-year-old man was complaining of progressive weight loss, which had been occurring for the past ten years, decreased strength, flatulence, and post-nasal drip. He had been losing weight for twelve years, had been worked up by numerous physicians without any relief, and had dropped to a low of 139 pounds, which bordered on undernutrition. None of the doctors who evaluated him over the last decade were able to explain why his health was degenerating. They also could offer him no help.

Not only did his MetaCT 400 test results revealed the underlying causes of all of his symptoms, such as weight loss, depression, feeling of quick fullness when eating, and gas and bloating. It also found major risk factors for other diseases, such as cardiovascular disease and dementia, all of which were corrected using targeted nutrient therapy. Specifically, the data showed: (1) food intolerances to milk and casein (a protein found in dairy); (2) fungal and bacterial dysbiosis; (3) deficiencies in all ten essential- and many non-essential amino acids; (4) elevated cardiovascular risk factors including fibrinogen and homocysteine; (5) multiple low minerals; (6) lead toxicity; (7) low omega-3 essential fatty acids; (8) multiple functional vitamin deficiencies; (9) low antioxidant status; (10) impaired liver detoxification pathways.

Multiple, severe amino acid deficiencies. In such cases the body will break down muscle protein, so repleting amino acids is crucial to correcting this condition.			
Arginine	51	50 - 160	
Histidine	65 L	70 - 140	
Isoleucine	43 L	50 - 160	
Leucine	76 L	90 - 200	
Lysine	134 L	150 - 300	
Methionine	24 L	25 - 50	
Phenylalanine	45	45 - 140	
Threonine	82 L	100 - 250	

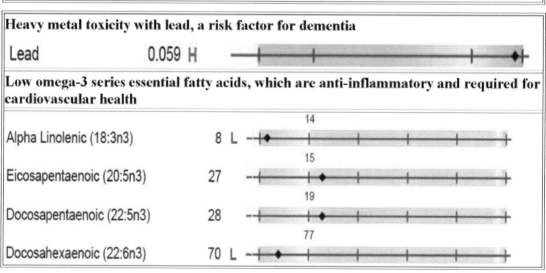

Tryptophan	35	35 - 65	
Valine	135 L	170 - 420	
Glycine	212 L	225 - 450	
Serine	74 L	90 - 210	
Taurine	43 L	50 - 250	
Tyrosine	41 L	50 - 120	

Low and low-normal essential minerals

Chromium	0.29	
Copper	0.53	
Magnesium	48	
Manganese	0.23 L	
Potassium	1,759	
Selenium	0.14	
Vanadium	0.11	
Zinc	6.4	

Heavy metal toxicity with lead, a risk factor for dementia

Lead	0.059 H	

Low omega-3 series essential fatty acids, which are anti-inflammatory and required for cardiovascular health

Alpha Linolenic (18:3n3)	8 L	
Eicosapentaenoic (20:5n3)	27	
Docosapentaenoic (22:5n3)	28	
Docosahexaenoic (22:6n3)	70 L	

Decreased ability to use fats to produce energy (functional deficiencies in carnitine and vitamin B2)

Suberate	5.0 H	3.4
Ethylmalonate	6.3 H	5.5

Decreased ability to use sugars (carbohydrates) to produce energy (functional deficiencies in lipoic acid, vitamins B1, B3, chromium and CoQ10)

Pyruvate	4.6 H	4.1
Lactate	21.40 H	19.4

Impaired liver detoxification pathways from toxic exposure

Glucarate	8.5 H	7.0
a-Hydroxybutyrate	1.3 H	1.2
Pyroglutamate	51	60
Sulfate	172	166 390

Intestinal bacterial overgrowth, likely causing malabsorption (decreased absorption) of nutrients and nutritional deficiencies

Phenylacetate	0.14 H	0.11
Phenylpropionate	0.3	2.1
p-Hydroxybenzoate	1.1 H	1.0
p-Hydroxyphenylacetate	23 H	15
Indican	86 H	81
Tricarballylate	1.3	1.6

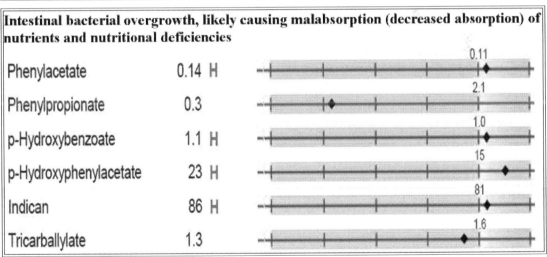

Intestinal fungal overgrowth, likely causing malabsorption (decreased absorption) of nutrients and nutritional deficiencies			
D-Arabinitol	45 H		

Allergies to milk, dairy, dairy products and products containing the protein *casein*.			
Casein	697	Mod	+4
Milk	671	Mod	+4

He was placed on a Targeted Nutritional Program to correct his nutritional deficiencies, which included a customized amino acid powder and specific blends of vitamins, minerals, and fatty acids. His intestinal infections were treated using antibacterial and antifungal agents. He followed a gut restoration protocol to repair any damage to his intestines that the infections might have caused, and he began a series of intravenous chelation treatments under the care of Dr. Neustadt in his clinic. His post-nasal drip cleared up, his strength increased, and his weight also went up to 149 pounds.

It is important to note here the very serious nature of his condition, which would have inevitably resulted in him being incapacitated and likely suffering an early death.

Treatment Plan

Diet:
AVOID all *milk, casein, and milk products for* eight weeks. See the handout on alternatives to milk products.

Exercise: Continue to work with your trainer on exercise, but ensure you are focusing on range of motion exercises and not weight-bearing exercises for one month. You may resume the weight-bearing exercises, albeit at moderate intensity, in one month.

For fungal infection in the intestines:
NYSTATIN TABLETS, 500,000 units twice daily for three months for this.

For bacterial overgrowth in the intestines:
BERBERINE FORTE: Take one capsule twice daily with food.

ENTEROPRO: Take one capsule daily with food.

For low amino acids:

RESCULPT: Stir or blend two two scoops (23g) of ReSculpt into 8 fl. oz. of water, milk, or juice *twice* daily. After one month, decrease your dosage to two scoops *once* daily.

L-HISTIDINE 600 mg: Take two capsules daily with a full glass of water or fruit or vegetable juice.

GLYCINE POWDER: Mix ½ teaspoon daily with water with or between meals.

TAURINE POWDER: Take 1/2 teaspoon daily on an empty stomach (thirty minutes before eating or 1.5 hours after eating).

GLUTAMINE RX: Mix one teaspoon twice daily in water and drink.

For elevated fibrinogen:

NATTOPINE: Take two capsules daily.

For functional vitamin deficiencies and low minerals:

SUPREME MULTIVITAMIN (WITHOUT IRON): Take four capsules daily with a meal.

PROMINERALS: Take three capsules daily with food. *Take one bottle and then discontinue.*

AN-30: Take one capsule twice daily with a meal.

MITOFORTE: Take four capsules with breakfast and maintain this higher dosage.

COFACTOR B: Take one capsule daily with food.

REJUVAMAG: Take two capsules each night before bed.

For elevated free radical damage:

VITAMIN C POWDER: Mix two scoops twice daily in water, and drink with a meal.

PROTECT DM: Take one capsule daily.

For lead toxicity:

CALCIUM-DISODIUM-EDTA INTRAVENOUS THERAPY

For low essential fatty acids:

CARLSON'S COD LIVER OIL: Take one *tablespoon* (equivalent of three teaspoons) daily for one month, then decrease your dose to two *teaspoons once daily.*

For low sulfur:

N-ACETYL-CYSTEINE (NAC) 1,000 mg: Take one capsule daily with food.

Chapter Nine

Osteoporosis

Osteoporosis is a major health concern in the United States and globally. According to US data obtained by the National Health and Nutrition Examination Survey (NHANES III, 1988-1994), 13% to 18% of women (4-6 million) over the age of 50 had osteoporosis, and 37% to 50% (13-17 million) had osteopenia.[117] Additionally, the estimated prevalence in men was 3% to 6% (1-2 million) for osteoporosis and 28% to 47% (8-13 million) for osteopenia. In the intervening years, the overall prevalence of osteoporosis has increased. In 2004, more than ten million people in the United States had been diagnosed with osteoporosis,[118] a number that by 2020 is projected to increase to fourteen million diagnosed cases.[119]

Osteoporosis is classified as either primary or secondary. Primary osteoporosis occurs with bone loss as people age, while secondary is caused by other factors such as medications (eg, glucocorticoids) and medical conditions (eg, Cushing's disease, hypogonadism, malabsorption).[120] Debilitating acute and chronic pain in the elderly is often attributed to fractures from osteoporosis and can lead to further disability and early mortality.[121, 122] In Caucasian women and men aged 50 years or older, the remaining lifetime risk of a hip, spine, or forearm fracture is estimated at 40% and 13%, respectively.[123] A 2005 report estimated that of the nearly two million osteoporosis fractures in the United States that year, 27% were vertebral fractures, 19% were wrist fractures, 14% were hip fractures, 7% were pelvic fractures, and 33% were "other" fractures. Nonvertebral fractures represented 73% of total fractures, with 71% of all fractures occurring in women.[119] It is startling to note that 12% to 40% of patients with osteoporosis who suffer hip fractures die within 6 months.[124] A 2009 article in *JAMA* concluded that the risk for death after a hip fracture is increased even five to ten years after the event.[125]

In addition to deleterious impacts on health, the economic effect of osteoporosis is significant and growing. In 2005 the cost for treating the more-than two million osteoporotic fractures in this country was almost $16.9 billion.[119] Of that, the largest cost ($12.8 billion) was spent on treating fractures in women, largely because they suffer a greater number of hip fractures than men (73% vs 69%, respectively). Although only 14% of all osteoporotic fractures were of the hip in 2005, they accounted for 72% of the total costs of treating osteoporotic fractures. By 2025 the estimated cost of treating more than 3 million expected fractures is projected to increase more than 48% to $25.3 billion.

Osteoporosis is generally viewed as a disease of low bone mineral density (BMD). This observation was first noted in 1940 when Fuller Albright, MD, of Massachusetts General Hospital observed decreased bone mass in ovariectomized pigeons.[126] In 1994 the World Health Organization (WHO) codified this paradigm by creating the official diagnosis of osteoporosis as having low BMD as defined by a "T" score. A T-score is a number of standard deviations from peak bone mass of healthy men or women, as appropriate, aged 20 to 29. A T-score of -2.5 or less is diagnostic of osteoporosis, while a T-score of -1 to -2.5 is diagnostic of osteopenia.

However, one of the reasons for this article is that T-score, and, hence, BMD, criteria may not accurately reflect fracture risk. In a longitudinal observational study, BMD tests were conducted at peripheral sites on postmenopausal women of 50 years or older (mean age 64.5 ± 9.3 years; range 50-104 years) without a previous diagnosis of osteoporosis.[127] Each woman received a baseline, in-office BMD test on the heel using single x-ray absorptiometry, forearm using peripheral dual-energy x-ray absorptiometry (DEXA), or finger using peripheral DEXA. Twelve months later participants completed a questionnaire asking if they had suffered any fractures since the study began and, if so, at which sites. While the fracture rates were, indeed, highest in women with the lowest T-scores, 82% of women who reported fractures of the wrist, forearm, hip, rib, or spine had a peripheral T-score greater than -2.5, and 67% had T-scores greater than -2.0. That is, the majority of fractures occurred in women who did *not* have a diagnosis of osteoporosis. A second study concluded that at age 50 years, the 10-year risk for fractures of the hip, spine, forearm, or proximal humerus in women with osteoporosis is approximately 45%; however, the study found 96% of all fractures in those locations occur in women without osteoporosis.[128]

Admittedly, bone density scans of the wrist, forearm and ribs are not standard. Dual-energy x-ray absorptiometry (DXA) is the current gold standard test for diagnosing osteoporosis in people without a known osteoporotic fracture. It is, however, an imperfect test, identifying less than one half of the people who progress to have an osteoporotic fracture. For example, in the Rotterdam Study, the sensitivity of DXA-determined osteoporosis was only 44% and 21% in identifying elderly women and men, respectively, who subsequently had a nonvertebral fracture.[129] Clearly, factors other than low bone mass are important in identifying patients at elevated risk for osteoporotic fracture.

Thus, if we are too reliant on the idea that BMD/T-scores vary consistently with fracture risk, we may fail to recognize danger signs and prevent painful, costly, and life-shortening fractures in patients. Early detection and treatment of risk factors for osteoporosis and osteoporotic fractures are essential for practicing clinicians. Family physicians will frequently be the doctors who recommend screening for osteoporosis and who are uniquely positioned to ensure both detection and appropriate treatment. Understanding bone histology, the physiology of bone turnover, and current research on the prevention and treatment of osteoporotic fractures can contribute towards the development of an integrative approach to treating this condition.

Factors That Influence Bone

During childhood and throughout puberty, the rate of bone creation is faster than the rate of bone loss; therefore, bones become larger and stronger. Bones continue to grow from birth until somewhere between the ages of 30 to 35.[130] Once peak bone mass has been achieved in the early 30s, men and women begin to lose bone at 0.5% to 2% per year, with considerable individual variation in the rate of bone loss.[131, 132] In women, an accelerated rate of loss occurs during menopause and for about 10 years thereafter.[133] As people of both sexes age, the risk of osteoporosis and of osteoporotic fractures increases.

Thus, we have come to realize that the skeleton that supports us does not stop changing once we've reached our full growth. Beyond natural aging factors, drugs, diet, and our own activities all have a continuing influence, for better or worse, on our bony structure.

The Osteoporotic Effects of Drugs, Cortisol, and Cadmium Toxicity

Glucocorticoids—including cortisone, prednisone, hydrocortisone, dexamethasone, and methylprednisolone—can all cause osteoporosis. Systemic corticosteroid use, such as of oral prednisone, for more than 6 months has been found to increase the risk for osteoporosis.[134, 135] One major reason for this is likely that corticosteroids modulate the immune system toward production of tumor necrosis factor-alpha, a marker of inflammation that stimulates bone resorption.[136]

Even very small doses of oral glucocorticoids (< 2.5 mg/day over approximately 6 months) are associated with a 20% to 200% increase in risk of vertebral fractures.[137] And for each 10 mg increase in dosage between patients, there was a 62% increase in risk for bone fracture.[138] This risk may be necessary and acceptable to control a disease process. However, if there are ways to reduce or halt the dosage of corticosteroids it would be advisable, since the risk for fracture decreases after stopping the medication.[137] If patients must take corticosteroid drugs, its deleterious effects on bone density may be reduced by supplementation with 45 mg per day of vitamin K_2 (as MK4).[139, 140]

The body's own production of cortisol can also contribute to osteoporosis. People with Cushing's disease, a rare condition in which the body produces excessively high, uncontrolled amounts of cortisol, are at an increased risk for osteoporosis and bone fractures. Two recent studies have shown that even normal, healthy people can also be producing enough cortisol to negatively affect bone. In one study of 34 "healthy" men ages 61 to 72 years, bone density was inversely correlated with cortisol levels.[141]

While not typically mentioned in conventional texts on osteoporosis, cadmium toxicity is also a risk factor. Tobacco smoke is one of the most common routes of exposure to cadmium, though it is also found in high amounts in food grown in contaminated soil, and in fish and shellfish caught from polluted water. At high doses, cadmium is toxic to the kidneys, which decreases the body's ability to make active vitamin D.[142] Producing less vitamin D decreases the ability to absorb dietary calcium and the body reacts by taking calcium from bones and other tissues such as muscles and nerves to use in the blood stream. Chronic exposure to even small amounts of cadmium can decrease bone mineral density[143, 144] by directly disrupting the balance between bone formation and destruction.[145] The most useful diagnostic test for cadmium exposure is a 24-hour urinary cadmium excretion standardized for creatinine. Even as little as 1 mcg cadmium per gram of creatinine has been associated with decreased bone density.[144]

Dietary Influences

Poor diet also increases cortisol. The standard Western diet with its high meat proteins and low fruit and vegetable intake acidifies the blood and increases cortisol. When an acidic diet is eaten long-term, chronically elevated cortisol may contribute to the known osteoporosis-promoting effects of this nutritional spectrum.[146] The intricate relationship between diet and bone health is still being untangled, but what is beyond dispute is that diet affects bone health.

One of the reasons that a meat-dense diet is problematic is that methionine, a sulfur-containing amino acid found in high concentrations in animal protein, can be converted in the body to homocysteine, a homologue of the naturally-occurring amino acid cysteine. Homocysteine interrupts the proper formation of collagen,[147] the main protein in bone and joints, which leads to bone degradation. But in addition to its bone-destroying effect, homocysteine directly damages blood vessels[148] and also reduces levels of glutathione, an important antioxidant.[149] Not only is homocysteine an independent risk factor for osteoporotic hip fractures,[21, 147] it is also a risk factor for cardiovascular disease.[150]

According to several studies, coffee (whether caffeinated or decaffeinated was not specified in the studies) can increase calcium excretion in the urine; however, this does not occur if people consume the dietary reference intakes (DRIs) or more of calcium per day.[151, 152] Interestingly, another study analyzed both diet and coffee consumption and the risk of fractures. It was conducted in Norway and more than 40 000 men and women, ages 47 to 68 years, participated. Only in women consuming a diet high in non-dairy animal protein and low in calcium was the risk for fractures increased. Women drinking 9 or more cups of coffee per day combined with low calcium intake also were at increased risk. The study concluded that, when drunk in moderation and in combination with a healthy diet and adequate calcium intake, coffee does not appear to increases one's risk for osteoporosis.[153]

Exercise

Not participating in routine aerobic, weight-bearing, and resistance exercises increases the risk of osteoporosis, broken bones, and an early death.[154-158] Appropriate exercise may prevent the onset of osteoporosis and has also been shown to increase BMD and decrease fracture risk. One year of weight-bearing exercise training in community-living women (ages 66 to 87 years) improved Ward's triangle BMD by 8.4% (P<.01) compared to controls.[159] Additionally, exercise can increase muscle mass, strength, and balance, thereby decreasing the risk for falling and suffering an osteoporotic fracture.[160] Muscle strengthening and balance exercises (eg, Chi Gong, Tai Chi) have been shown to decrease risk for fall and fall-related injuries by 75% among women aged 75 years and older.[161]

Integrative Clinical Approaches

As mentioned earlier, family physicians will frequently be the doctors who recommend screening for osteoporosis and who are uniquely positioned to ensure early detection and appropriate treatment.

In forestalling fractures, reducing risk for falling is crucial, as are implementing strategies that have been shown in clinical trials to significantly reduce fracture risk. Encouraging appropriate exercise and counseling patients to optimize their diet is also appropriate. However, exercise and dietary changes may be difficult in the elderly if they are unable to cook for themselves, have dementia, or have no independent means of transportation.

Assessing Fracture Risk

The large number of risk factors for osteoporosis can make clinical decision-making difficult. If all of these risk factors were given equal importance, practically everyone would be getting a DEXA scan. Although a full evaluation of the relative risks for each of these risk factors is beyond the scope of this review, several useful tools are available.

ACOG: In January 2004, the American College of Obstetricians and Gynecologists (ACOG) published its guidelines for osteoporosis screening. In that document it recommend BMD testing (1) should be advised for all postmenopausal women 65 years old or older; (2) may be recommended to postmenopausal women less than 65 years old with one or more risk factors for osteoporosis (see Table 9.1 for risk factors); and (3) should be performed on all postmenopausal women with fractures (whether previous or current fractures was not specified, but clinically, it would be good practice to look at both).

Table 9.1. ACOG Risk Factors for Osteoporosis[155]

Medical History That Increases Risk
History of prior fracture
Family history of osteoporosis
Caucasian race
Dementia
Poor nutrition
Smoking
Low weight and body mass index (BMI)
Estrogen deficiency resulting from • early menopause (age younger than 45 years) or bilateral oophorectomy • prolonged premenopausal amenorrhea (>1 year)
Long-term low calcium intake
Alcoholism
Impaired eyesight
History of falls
Inadequate physical activity
Medical Conditions That Increase Risk
Acquired immunodeficiency syndrome or human immunodeficiency virus
Amyloidosis
Ankylosing spondylitis
Chronic obstructive pulmonary disease
Congenital porphyria
Cushing's disease
Eating disorders
Female athlete triad (disordered eating, amenorrhea, and osteoporosis)
Gastrectomy
Gaucher's disease
Hemochromatosis
Hemophilia
Hyperparathyroidism
Hypogonadism, primary and secondary
Hypophosphatasia
Idiopathic scoliosis
Inadequate diet
Inflammatory bowel disease

| Insulin-dependent diabetes mellitus |
| Lymphoma and leukemia |
| Malabsorption syndromes (eg, lactose intolerance) |
| Mastocytosis |
| Multiple myeloma |
| Multiple sclerosis |
| Pernicious anemia |
| Rheumatoid arthritis |
| Severe liver disease, especially primary biliary cirrhosis |
| Spinal cord transaction |
| Sprue |
| Stroke (cerebrovascular accident) |
| Thalassemia |
| Thyrotoxicosis |
| Tumor secretion of parathyroid hormone-related peptide |
| Weight loss |
| **Medications That Increase Risk** |
| Aluminum (eg, aluminum-containing antacids) |
| Anticonvulsants (phenobarbital, phenytoin) |
| Cytotoxic drugs |
| Glucocorticosteroids and adrenocorticotropin |
| Gonadotropin-releasing hormone agonists |
| Heparin (long-term use) |
| Immunosupressants |
| Lithium |
| Progesterone, parenteral, long-acting |
| Tamoxifen (premenopausal use) |
| Thyroxine (at supraphysiologic doses) |
| Total parenteral nutrition |
| **Additional Risks** |
| Cadmium toxicity[136] |
| Endogenous, non-pathological cortisol production[134] |
| Low antioxidant status[156] |

WHO: Two years prior to the publication of the ACOG guidelines, J.A. Kanis, of the WHO Collaborating Centre for Metabolic Bone Disease at the University of Sheffield Medical School in England, published an evaluation of the 10-year risk of osteoporotic fractures.[128] He concluded that factors other than low BMD increase the risk for fractures. These factors include age, previous fragility fractures, glucocorticoid therapy, high bone turnover, family history of hip fracture, low bodyweight, neuromuscular disorders, cigarette smoking, and poor visual acuity (if someone can't see well, they're more likely to bump into something and/or misstep and fall, thereby increasing there risk for fracture). In fact, a history of a previous fall is a greater indicator for fracture risk than is BMD alone because a previous fall indicates the potential a future fall, which is a risk for fracture.[164]

NAMS: In 2006 the North American Menopause Society (NAMS) published a position statement on managing osteoporosis.[120] It concluded that fracture risk "depends largely on factors other than BMD." Combining a BMD with a physical examination (discussed below) and risk factors for osteoporotic fractures (see Table 9.2) provide a more comprehensive risk assessment. The NAMS guidelines also take falling into account and provide some practical and relatively inexpensive suggestions for decreasing falling risk, which clinicians can easily discuss with patients (see Table 9.3).

Table 9.2. NAMS Risk Factors for Osteoporotic Fractures[113]

Advanced age
Low bone mineral density (BMD)
Previous fracture (other than skull, facial bone, ankle, finger, or toe as an adult)
History of hip fracture in a parent
Thinness (body weight < 127 lbs [57.7 kg] or low BMI [<21 kg/m^2])
Current smoking, any amount
Low calcium or vitamin D intake
More than two alcoholic drinks per day
Oral or intramuscular glucocorticoid use for >3 months
Increased fall risk from: <ul><li>Impaired vision</li><li>Dementia</li><li>Poor health/frailty</li><li>Low physical activity</li><li>History of recent falls</li></ul>

Table 9.3. NAMS Recommendations for Fall Prevention[113]

Lighting • Provide ample lighting • Have easy-to-locate light switches for rooms and stairs • Use night lights to illuminate walkways
Obstructions • Remove clutter, low-lying objects • Remove raised door sills to ensure smooth transition
Floors and carpets • Provide nonskid rugs on slippery floors • Repair/replace worn, buckled, or curled carpet • Use nonskid floor wax
Furniture • Arrange furniture to ensure clear pathways • Remove or avoid low chairs and armless chairs • Adjust bed height if too high or low
Storage • Install shelves and cupboards at accessible height • Keep frequently used items at waist height
Bathroom • Install grab bars in tub, shower, near toilet • Use chair in shower and tub • Install nonskid strips/decals in tub/shower • Elevate low toilet seat or install safety frame
Stairways and halls • Install handrails on both sides of stairs • Remove or tape down throw rugs and runners • Repair loose and broken steps • Install nonskid treads on steps

The Fracture-Risk Assessment Tool

Fortunately for clinical decision-making, WHO has aggregated the data and created a free, online clinical-assessment tool called the Fracture-Risk Assessment Tool, or FRAX. This easy-to-use application provides a 10-year probability of fractures given a person's ethnicity, body mass index, medical history, and age. FRAX can be accessed at http://www.shef.ac.uk/FRAX/index.htm. This tool can help clinicians decide quickly with whom they should implement therapies to reduce fracture risk.

Physical Exam

While no single physical examination finding, or combination of findings, can rule in osteoporosis or spinal fracture without further testing, a physical examination can raise or lower clinical suspicion and provide important data as to the strength of a recommendation for further evaluation.

Some pieces to consider:

Thoracic Fracture: An occult thoracic fracture may be suspected if the measured distance from the wall to the a patient's occiput (Wall-Occiput Distance) is greater than zero centimeters when they are standing with their heals touching the wall.[165]

Lumbar Fracture: An occult lumbar fracture may be suspected if the distance between the inferior margin of the ribs and the iliac crest, called the Rib-Pelvis Distance, is less than two fingerbreadths.[165]

Height Loss: A 2005 study by Kerry Siminoski, MD, and colleagues from the University of Alberta, Edmonton, Canada, evaluated the relationship between height loss and vertebral-fracture risk in 985 postmenopausal women.[166] Dr Siminoski concluded that a height loss of greater than 2.0 cm over 3 years was 35.5% sensitive and 93.6% specific for detecting new fractures when compared against radiographic morphometry.

Physical Characteristics: Osteoporosis risk also increases if a person has fewer than 20 teeth because this may indicate bone resorption in the jaw, which may indicate body-wide bone resorption and osteoporosis. It also increases if a person has a self-reported kyphosis, or weighs less than 51 kg (approximately 112 pounds).[165] For a list of these physical examination risk factors, see Table 9.4.

Table 9.4. Physical examination maneuvers suggesting presence of osteoporosis or spinal fractures[158, 159]

Wall-Occiput Distance
Inability to touch occiput to the wall when standing with back and heels to the wall
Weight
Less than 51 kg (approximately 112 pounds)
Height
Loss of ≤ 2.0 cm over 1-3 years
Rib-Pelvis Distance
Less than 2 fingerbreadths between the inferior margin of the ribs and the superior surface of the pelvis in the midaxillary line
Tooth Count
Fewer than 20 teeth
Self-reported Humped Back
Patient report that back has become humped

Pharmacological Therapies

Pharmacological therapy is the standard of care for conventional approaches to osteoporosis treatment. Antiresorptive pharmacological therapies, such as alendronate (Fosamax), risedronate (Actonel), raloxifene (Evista), and parathyroid hormone minimally improve BMD. They have also been shown to effectively decrease vertebral fracture risk by 47% for alendronate,[167] 49% for risendronate,[168] 30% for raloxifene,[169] and 65% for parathyroid hormone[170] (see Table 9.5). However, some studies have concluded that with antiresorptive drug therapies BMD accounts for only 4% to 28% of the reduction in vertebral fracture risk.[171-174] Thus, focusing solely on therapies that increase BMD does not maximize potential clinical benefits.

Additionally, new evidence is suggesting that treatment with bisphosphonate medications may actually increase fracture risk after approximately seven years of use. A recent retrospective review of patients admitted to a Level 1 trauma center over a five-year period was published in the *Journal of Orthopaedic Trauma*.[175] During that time period, 70 patients (59 women, 11 men; mean age 74.7 years) were evaluated. Twenty-five of these patients had been taking alendronate, and of those 25, there were 19 (76%) who experienced a "transverse facture with a unicortical break in an area of cortical hypertrophy." In contrast, only 1 patient (2%)

not being treated with alendronate suffered this fracture pattern. The odd ratio of a fracture for people taking alendronate was 139.33 (*P*<.0001). The average duration of alendronate treatment was significantly greater in those with the fracture pattern compared those without this pattern: 6.9 years versus 2.5 years, respectively (*P*=.002).

At least two additional retrospective analyses have come to similar conclusions. One study published in *The Journal of Bone and Joint Surgery Br* identified thirteen women who suffered subtrochanteric fractures with minimal or no trauma over a 10-month period from May 2005 to February 2006 in two hospitals in Singapore.[176] Of those women, nine had been taking alendronate for an average of 4.2 years (2.5 to 5.0 years; mean age 66.9 years), and four had not been taking alendronate. Interestingly, of these 13, there were 4 who reported a BMD score that put them in the category of osteopenia rather than osteoporosis. Three others reported BMD scores that placed them in the osteoporosis category and the rest did not report a score.

Another report of US cases is particularly condemning: The report identified 9 patients who experienced traumatic nonspinal fractures after 3 to 8 years of alendronate therapy "while performing normal daily activities such as walking, standing, or turning around."[177] These patients continued taking alendronate after their fracture and 6 of those patients exhibited delayed fracture healing for 3 months to 2 years after the fracture.

While preliminary, these reports are alarming. There is evidence that alendronate therapy may suppress bone remodeling to the point of increasing fracture risk in some patients. This risk may be extremely small, but no long-term prospective study has been carried out to quantify this risk. In the meantime, clinicians may consider other medication and/or a more integrative approach than monotherapy with alendronate to help decrease fracture risk in their patients.

Nutritional Therapies

One of the conceptual problems with many clinical trials of dietary supplements for BMD or fracture prevention is that they tend to study effects of only 1 or maybe 2 added nutrients. However, bone is a complex mixture of different minerals, and even minerals that are not found in the bone matrix are still required as cofactors in bone remodeling. The importance of vitamin and mineral supplements in maintaining bone health was demonstrated in a study of postmenopausal women ages 50 to 60.[178] Those women who took a complex supplement containing calcium, magnesium, zinc, and vitamins D and K lost significantly less BMD than those who did not take the supplement.

Calcium and Vitamin D

Calcium and vitamin D are currently recommended for the primary prevention of osteoporosis and the primary and secondary prevention of osteoporotic fractures. Secondary prevention of osteoporotic fracture was assessed in a trial of 5292 people aged 70 years or older (mean age, 77 years).[179] Volunteers (85% female) were randomized to receive 1 of 4 protocols: 800 IU vitamin D_3, 1000 mg calcium carbonate, 800 IU vitamin D_3 plus 1000 mg calcium carbonate, or placebo daily for up to 62 months (median duration, 45 months). In this trial no significant difference in fracture risk was detected between groups.

However, another study noted a 16% reduction in fracture risk ($P < .025$) over 3 years in 2532 community-dwelling residents (median age, 73 years; 59.8% female) who supplemented with 400 IU vitamin D_3 and 1000 mg calcium as calcium carbonate daily.[180] As well, in a randomized, open-label, 2-year sequential follow-up study of 43 healthy adult volunteers (14 men, mean age 60.6 years; 29 postmenopausal women, mean age 54.1 years), participants followed their usual diet for the first year and then were randomized to receive 500 IU vitamin D_3 and 500 mg calcium (form of calcium not reported), or no supplementation, from October to March.[181] During these winter months in which volunteers took vitamin D_3 and calcium, their lumbar BMD was 0.8% greater than in controls ($P=.04$), while no significant differences between the groups were noted for femoral-neck BMD.

Vitamin K_2

Vitamin K is a group of structurally similar, lipid-soluble, 2-methyl-1,4-napthoquinones, which include phylloquinone (K_1), menaquinones (K_2) and menadione (K_3).[110] Plants synthesize vitamin K_1 while bacteria can produce a range of vitamin K_2 forms, including the conversion of K_1 to K_2 by bacteria in the small intestines. Vitamin K_3 is synthetic and, because of its toxicity, has been banned in by the US Food and Drug Administration for human uses. In contrast to vitamin K_3, no known toxicity exists for the vitamin K_1 and K_2 forms.

Taking broad-spectrum antibiotics can reduce vitamin K production in the gut by nearly 74% in people compared to those not taking these antibiotics.[182] Diets low in vitamin K also decrease the body's vitamin K concentration.[183] Additionally, in the elderly there is a reduction in vitamin K_2 production.[184] Natto (fermented soybean) is the richest dietary source of vitamin K_2. Dairy products (milk, butter, cottage cheese, cheese) and egg yolk also provide small amounts.

It's important to note that vitamin K_1 is preferentially used by the liver as a clotting factor. Vitamin K_2 on the other hand is used preferentially in other organs, such as the brain, vasculature, breasts and kidneys. Coagulation studies in humans using 45 mg per day of vitamin K_2 (as MK4)[105] and even up to 135 mg/day (45 mg tid) of K_2 (as MK4),[107] showed no significant increase in pathologic coagulation risk. Even doses in rats as high as 250 mg/kg body weight did not alter the tendency for blood-clot formation to occur.[108]

Clinicians should also understand that there are primarily two forms of vitamin K_2 commercially available. These are MK4 and MK7. MK4 is a synthetic form of vitamin K_2 and the agent used in the clinical trials mentioned below. MK7 is produced by bacterial fermentation of soy, appears to have a longer half life then MK4, and can also decrease serum ucOC.[111] However, only MK4 has demonstrated the ability to decrease fracture risk, the clinically relevant end point in randomized, controlled clinical trials.

Vitamin K_2 exerts a powerful influence on bone building, especially in osteoporosis, and in Japan has been accepted as an osteoporosis treatment.[102] It is a fat-soluble vitamin that is a coenzyme for a vitamin K-dependent carboxylase enzyme that catalyzes carboxylation of the amino acid glutamic acid, resulting in its conversion to gamma-carboxyglutamic acid (Gla). This carboxylation reaction is essential for formation of bone collagen, which allows bone to deform upon impact, for example during a fall, without fracturing. Although vitamin K-dependent gamma-carboxylation occurs only on specific glutamic acid residues in a small number of proteins, it is critical to the calcium-binding function of those proteins.

Three vitamin K-dependent proteins have been isolated in bone—osteocalcin, matrix Gla protein (MGP) and protein S. Osteocalcin is a protein that is synthesized by osteoblasts and is regulated by the active form of vitamin D, $1,25\text{-}(OH)_2D_3$, also called calcitriol. The mineral-binding capacity of osteocalcin requires vitamin K-dependent gamma-carboxylation of 3 glutamic acid residues. Multiple randomized, double-blind, placebo-controlled clinical trials have shown significant decreases in undercarboxylated osteocalcin (ucOC) in volunteers supplemented with 45 mg of vitamin K_2 with and without the addition of calcium and vitamin D_3 compared to controls.[103-106]

A 2006 meta-analysis published in the *Archives of Internal Medicine* by Sarah Cockayne, MSc, Joy Adams, PhD, Susan Lanham-New, PhD, and colleagues, at the University of York in England, evaluated clinical trials on vitamin K_2 and fracture risk.[109] They identified 13 randomized, controlled trials of the effect of vitamin K_2 on osteoporosis. Of those, 7 had fracture risk as an end point and so were included in their meta-analysis. They concluded that 45 mg of vitamin K_2 as menaquinone-4 (MK-4) could decrease vertebral fracture by 60%, hip fracture by 73%, and all nonvertebral fractures by 81%.

An excellent review of vitamin K_2 by Stephen Plaza, ND, and Davis Lamson, ND, was published in 2005 in the journal *Alternative Medicine Review*.[110] In this article they reviewed clinical trials using vitamin K_2 that showed increases in BMD and/or reduction in fracture risk in volunteers who had bone loss from anorexia nervosa, Parkinson's disease, biliary cirrhosis, and stroke and in volunteers who were taking prednisone and leuprolide; in other volunteers, it increased the efficacy of bisphosphonate medications.

Antioxidants

In healthy bone, free radicals are used by osteoclasts to "chisel away at older bone,"[185] which creates small holes in bone that are filled by osteoblasts with new bone. As long as this is kept in check, all is well. When the balance becomes skewed to too many free radicals, however, (ie, an inadequate intake of antioxidants) osteoporosis may result. An Italian study compared the antioxidant status of 75 post-menopausal, osteoporotic women to 75 women without osteoporosis, ages 62 to 79 years, for 12 months. Compared to controls, postmenopausal women with osteoporosis had significantly lower levels of plasma vitamin A (2.37 ± 0.22 vs 2.14 ± 0.22 µmol/L, respectively), plasma vitamin C (55.5 ± 13.1 vs 30 ± 3.7 µmol/L, respectively), plasma vitamin E (62.8 ± 8.76 vs 46.7 ± 5 µmol/L, respectively), plasma uric acid (383.5 ± 63.7 vs 227.8 ± 34.6 µmol/L, respectively), plasma glutathione peroxidase (0.11 ± 0.01 vs 0.09 ± 0.01 mmol NADPH/min/mil, respectively), plasma superoxide dismutase (31.34 ± 3.1 vs 24.22 ± 3.8 U/ml, respectively), and erythrocyte superoxide dismutase (3402 ± 505.8 vs 2265 ± 314.7 U/g hemoglobin, respectively).[163] All antioxidant concentrations correlated with femoral BMD; however, significant positive correlations were noted only for vitamin A ($P < .01$), vitamin C ($P < .05$), and plasma glutathione peroxidase ($P < .05$).

Previous human studies have shown that vitamin C supplementation, especially in conjunction with calcium supplementation, and vitamin E protect against bone loss.[186-188]

In an animal study, supplementation with N-acetylcysteine increased glutathione levels.[189] Although no randomized, controlled trial has been conducted that analyzed the effects of multi-antioxidant supplementation on bone health, it is logical to conclude that increasing the body's antioxidants may help decrease the rate of loss of BMD.

Other Micronutrients

Osteoporosis risk is increased by low intakes of calcium,[190, 191] potassium,[192] magnesium,[192] and vitamin K;[193] and by low concentrations of vitamin D.[191] Additionally, people with low BMD have lower zinc concentrations in their bones.[194] Copper and zinc are important for bone health. Zinc is found in the bone matrix incorporated into hydroxyapatite crystal. It is also involved in stimulating osteoblastic activity while suppressing osteoclastic activity.[195] Copper, also required for bone formation, is a cofactor for the lysyl-oxidase enzyme.[195] This enzyme forms collagen and elastin cross-links from the essential amino acid lysine.[195]

Strontium

Strontium, an alkaline earth metal, has been studied for it's ability to increase BMD and reduce fracture risk. Strontium ranelate (SR) is a form of strontium salt from ranelic acid patented by a French company. SR is well studied and currently approved for the treatment of osteoporosis in most of Europe but is not yet approved in the United States. Animal studies have shown it to have an affinity for bone, decreasing bone resorption and increasing bone formation in rats.[196] A recent in vitro study determined that SR affects bone through induction of osteoblastogenesis.[197] Several studies have evaluated the efficacy of SR in preventing and reversing osteoporosis in experimental animals and humans.

In 2002 results were published from a phase II, 2-year, randomized, multicenter, double-blind, placebo-controlled, dose-response trial of SR for the treatment of osteoporosis (STRATOS).[198] Participants in the study were 353 non-obese, post-menopausal, osteoporotic women between 45 and 78 years of age who were randomized to one of 4 groups (placebo, SR 0.5 g/d, SR 1.0 g/d, and SR 2.0 g/d). In addition to supplemental strontium or placebo, all patients received supplemental calcium (500 mg/d) and vitamin D (vitamin D_3, 800 IU/d) "to ensure," as the researchers said, "that patients affected by severe osteoporosis received a minimum level of active treatment." All women had at least 1 previous vertebral fracture (T4 to L5) and a lumbar T-score of -2.4 or less. The primary endpoint was lumbar BMD, and the secondary outcomes included femoral neck BMD (FN-BMD), incidence of new vertebral deformities, and biochemical markers of bone metabolism. Bone measurements were tested using DEXA and were verified by iliac crest bone biopsies taken at months 12 and 24.

An increase in BMD was observed in all treatment groups by 12 months, with further increases at 24 months. FN-BMD also increased in treatment groups, but decreased in the placebo group. By the end of the second year of the study, the incidence of new vertebral deformities, while having increased in the placebo group, decreased in the treatment groups. However, during the second year, women receiving 0.5 g SR/day had a 0.51 (95% CI 0.31; 0.84) relative risk of experiencing a new deformity, while women taking 2 g SR/day had a relative risk of 0.56 (95% CI 0.35; 0.89). The overall relative risk of a new deformity over the entire 2-year period, compared to placebo, was 0.71 (95% CI 0.49; 1.02) and 0.77 (95% CI 0.54; 1.09) in the SR 0.5 g/d and SR 2.0 g/d groups, respectively. Urinary excretion of bone-resorption markers was decreased in all treatment groups, while alkaline phosphatase (an indicator of osteoblast activity) was increased. Although the fracture risk was greater in the higher treatment group (2 g SR /d) versus the lower (0.5 g SR/day), the higher SR group experienced the greatest increases in BMD, about 3% per year. Adverse effects were mild to moderate, and the treatment was well tolerated in all treatment groups.

A second study evaluated the reduction in fracture risk in a phase III, randomized, double-blind, 3-year clinical trial utilizing 2 g SR/d or placebo in 1442 postmenopausal women (mean age approximately 69 years) with osteoporosis.[199] All volunteers also received at lunchtime, dependent on dietary calcium intake, up to 1000 mg elemental calcium to ensure an intake of more than 1500 mg calcium daily, plus 400 to 800 IU vitamin D (form of vitamin D not specified), depending on their baseline vitamin D_2 (25-hydroxyvitamin D) status.

After 12 months, total vertebral-fracture risk decreased by 49% in the SR group compared to placebo ($P<.001$), and the SR group also had a 52% reduction of symptomatic fractures ($P=.003$). By the end of the 3-year study, BMD in the SR group increased over baseline by 12.7% at the lumbar spine, 7.2% at the femoral neck, and 8.6% at the total hip ($P<.001$ for all three sites). Also by study end, volunteers taking SR had a 41% lower risk of a new vertebral fracture than those in the placebo group ($P<.001$). The researchers concluded that to prevent one patient from suffering a vertebral fracture, nine patients would need to be treated for three years with SR.

A cautionary note should be inserted about SR. Strontium has an atomic mass greater than calcium. As such it attenuates the X-rays from a DEXA scan to a greater extent than calcium.[198] Unless the radiologist corrects for this, the DEXA scan will not provide an accurate measure of BMD.[198] Additionally, the form of strontium used in clinical trials (strontium ranelate) is not available in the United States. The form available in dietary supplements in the US is strontium citrate. Although the strontium citrate form may be effective at improving BMD and decreasing fracture risk, clinical trials have not been performed on strontium citrate to demonstrate its safety and efficacy.

Table 9.5. Reduction in risk of fracture

Drug/Dietary Supplement	Percent risk reduction and site
Alendronate (Fosamax) 10 mg[160]	47%, all vertebra
Risedronate (Actonel) 5 mg[161]	49%, all vertebra
Raloxifene (Evista) 60 mg[162]	30%, all vertebra
Parathyroid hormone 20 mcg to 40 mcg[163]	65% to 69%, respectively, all vertebra
Strontium ranelate 500-2000 mg[192]	41-49%, all vertebra
Vitamin K2 (as MK4) 45 mg [107]	60%, all vertebra, 73%, hip, 81% all nonvertebral fractures

Chapter Ten

Osteoarthritis

Osteoarthritis (OA) is a chronic, degenerative disease of articular cartilage. It usually occurs in the older age-group and is a nearly universal consequence of aging in vertebrates. Unlike some autoimmune diseases and cancer, OA is not a disease of modernity, although certain factors of modern environment (e.g., chronic stress and nutrient deficiencies) may contribute to its pathogenesis.

OA has been documented among prehistoric animals and is found in both reptiles and birds. OA occurred in ancient animals, fish, amphibians, reptiles (dinosaurs), birds, mammoths, and cave bears. It affects almost all vertebrates, suggesting that it appeared with the evolutionary arrival of the bony skeleton. It occurs in whales, dolphins, and porpoises, which are supported by water, but not in bats and sloths, which hang upside down. This suggests that OA is an ancient Paleozoic mechanism of repair and remodeling rather than a disease in the usual sense.[200] It also suggests that gravity and the steady mechanical forces upon the joint tissues are primary contributing factors.

Epidemiology

Arthritis is the leading cause of disability in the United States.[201] According for the Center for Disease Control (CDC), "Arthritis and related conditions affect nearly 43 million Americans, or about one of every six people, making it one of the most prevalent diseases nationally. By

2020, as the baby boom generation ages, an estimated 60 million Americans will be affected by arthritis." Currently over 40 million Americans have some form of degenerative joint disease, including 80% of people over fifty years old.[202]

Osteoarthritis increases with age, and sex-specific differences are evident. Before fifty years of age, the prevalence of OA in most joints is higher in men than in women. After about age fifty years, women are more often affected with hand, foot, and knee osteoarthritis than men. In most studies, hip osteoarthritis is more frequent in men.[203]

The physical evidence of OA first appears in the second and third decades of life, although the disease is usually asymptomatic until much later, typically the fifth or sixth decade. By the seventh decade, OA is nearly universal, producing the highest rate of morbidity of any disease.[202] Although primarily seen in the elderly, there is a 35% incidence in the knee as early as age thirty (often diagnosed as chondromalacia patellae).[204]

Rates of arthritis are higher in rural populations, and those with low education or low income. Rates are similar for whites (15.2%) and blacks (15.5%), but relatively low for Asian/ Pacific Islanders (7.3%) and Hispanics (11.3%). Rates among people in the northeast and western regions of the United States are lower than those among other regions.[205]

Pathophysiology

Osteoarthritis results from structural changes in the articular cartilage in the joints, usually those that are weight-bearing, such as the spine and knees. The OA disease process at the tissue and cellular level is associated with destruction and loss of cartilage, remodeling of bone, and intermittent inflammation.[206]

In the healthy adult joint there is a constant turnover of cells. As old, worn out cells are degraded, new healthy cells are produced. In the pathological state, this balance is disrupted, and the rate of degeneration is faster than the rate of repair. Ultimately, elevated matrix degradation results in complete loss of the cartilage and loss in joint function.

Articular cartilage that lines the surface of long bones is a multilayered material. The superficial layer consists of collagen fibrils and chondrocytes that run parallel to the joint surface. In the deeper layers, the collagen fibrils are more randomly arranged and support vertical units termed chondrons containing rows of chondrocytes. In the deepest layers, the collagen fibrils run almost vertically and ultimately insert into the underlying subchondral bone.

OA affects articular cartilage and is characterized by enzymatic and mechanical breakdown of the extracellular matrix, leading to cartilage degeneration, exposure of subchondral bone, pain, and limited joint motion.[207, 208]

Risk factors for developing osteoarthritis include age; previous joint injury; nutrient deficiency, particularly antioxidants; obesity; hormonal imbalances; environmental pollutants; poor lifestyle; and a genetic predisposition.[206, 209-212] An imbalance of joint functioning initiates the disease process, which is then worsened through biochemical changes in the collagen in the joint.[210]

Diagnosis

OA is diagnosed as primary (idiopathic) or secondary. In primary OA there is no identifiable other condition that caused the OA. Subsets of primary OA include erosive, inflammatory OA and rapidly destructive OA of the shoulders and less often of hips and knees.[200] Primary OA is sometimes referred to as "wear-and-tear osteoarthritis." In secondary OA, as the label implies, OA is a result of another condition, such as trauma, an autoimmune process, or structural abnormalities. Irrespective of the type of OA diagnosed, a metabolic dysfunction is occurring, and this underlying dysfunction must be addressed to optimize treatment.

There is no current "gold standard" for the diagnosis of osteoarthritis.[206] Radiographic and lab testing do not correlate well with the disease and joint pain is the cardinal clinical presentation.[210, 213] In fact, the frequent dissociation between change in joint structure and occurrence of symptoms suggests that many first-time patients who seek medical care for joint pain will already have advanced destruction of their joint cartilage.[206]

Diagnosis is usually made based on clinical presentation. The chief symptoms of osteoarthritis are pain and stiffness in the joints. It most often affects asymmetrical weight bearing joints and distal interphalangeal (DIP) joints. The pain usually increases after exercise. Other symptoms may include watery eyes, dry neck, leg cramps, allergies, arteriosclerosis, impairment in the functioning of the gall-bladder and liver disturbances.

Treatment

Because of the chronic nature of osteoarthritis, nonpharmacologic interventions can provide patients self-care strategies that may lessen pain, improve physical functioning, and increase independence and sense of control. Nonpharmacologic interventions include exercise, rest and joint protection, heat and cold, hydrotherapy, therapeutic touch, acupuncture/acupressure, biofeedback, hypnotherapy, cognitive-behavioral techniques, activity and home maintenance modification, nutrition, and transportation interventions.[214]

The therapeutic approach recommended here is remove stressors and rebalance the body. To this end, the goals include reducing joint stress and trauma, promoting collagen repair mechanisms, eliminating allergic foods and other factors that may inhibit normal collagen repair, optimizing digestion and absorption of nutrients, and clearing toxins from the body. All diseases or predisposing factors should be controlled.

Non-steroidal anti-inflammatory drugs (NSAIDs), such as aspirin, acetaminophen, indomethacin, and diclofenac, should be avoided as much as possible. While effective at suppressing the symptoms of OA, chronic NSAID use may accelerate joint damage by enhancing the production of pro-inflammatory cytokines and inhibiting cartilage proteoglycan synthesis.[215]

Cross-linking of glycosaminoglycans (GAG) by sulfur is necessary for the production and stability of articular cartilage. Production of articular cartilage is very senstive to even slight fluctuations in sulfur concentrations. Van der Kraan et al[216] showed that a 0.1 mM decrease in serum sulfate concentration resulted in a 33% decrease in GAG production. Aspirin and sodium salicylates inhibit the incorporation of sulfur into proteoglycans *in vitro.*[217] Additionally, acetominophen and other drugs metabolized by hepatic sulfation have been shown to deplete the body's sulfate reserves.[218, 219]

One therapeutic strategy includes the use methylsulfonylmethane (MSM) as a sulfur donor. NSAIDs may decrease MSMs therapeutic effect by using up MSM in the liver for NSAID detoxification rather than for GAG cross-linking in the joints.

If aspirin or other NSAIDs must be used, deglycyrrhizinated licorice root (*Glycyrrhiza glabra*) and/or glutamine powder can be used to help protect the gastrointestinal tract from its damaging effects, and its use should be discontinued as soon as possible. Data from epidemiologic studies show that among persons sixty-five years of age or older, 20% to 30% of all hospitalizations and deaths due to peptic ulcer disease were attributable to therapy with NSAIDs.[220]

Lifestyle

As in all chronic degenerative diseases, lifestyle plays a major role in its onset and progression. Adequate sleep and stress reduction are crucial. Human growth hormone (HGH) is critical for tissue repair, and the body secretes the most HGH during the deepest stage of sleep. The necessity of getting adequate quality *and* quantity of sleep cannot be understated.

Inadequate sleep also puts stress on the body. This, combined with a stressful lifestyle, increases the adrenal glands' production of cortisol. Cortisol decreases HGH secretion[221] and thus inhibits the body's own repair mechanisms.

Hydrocortisone therapy is sometimes used in conventional medicine to treat the symptoms of osteoarthritis and other chronic pain syndromes. The problem is that cortisol and its derivatives inhibit cellular repair and regeneration.[222] Although it may dramatically decrease the pain initially, this therapy is of limited long-term value and may increase the progression of joint degeneration in OA.

Diet

Giving the body the raw materials it needs to regenerate damaged tissue can greatly speed recovery. The most important, and often overlooked, nutrient in the body is water. All cells in the body are bathed in water, and all joints use water as a shock absorber. Ensure that adequate amounts of clean water are consumed.

To get a rough estimate of how much water one should be drinking, divide the person's body weight by two. The resulting number is the amount of water, in ounces, that should be drunk each day. For example, a 160-pound person would want to shoot for eighty ounces of water a day, or approximately ten eight-ounce glasses. Caffeine is a diuretic and also depletes magnesium, B-vitamins, and other nutrients.

Six decades of conventional agriculture have depleted our nation's soils of important nutrients. Organic agriculture has significantly higher concentrations vitamin C, iron, magnesium, and phosphorus and significantly less nitrates than conventional agriculture.[223, 224] Worthington recently showed that there is a higher content of nutritionally significant minerals with lower amounts of some heavy metals in organic crops compared to conventional ones.[223] And in another study, animals fed organically grown feed had better growth and reproduction compared with those fed conventionally grown feed.[224]

Identify and avoid all intolerant or allergic foods. Eliminating nightshade vegetables (family Solanaceae), which includes tomatoes, potatoes, eggplant, peppers, and tobacco, may be helpful. Presumably, these alkaloids inhibit normal collagen repair in the joints or promote inflammatory degeneration of the joint.[225] This diet has been of benefit to some individuals and is certainly worth a try. People may react to other foods as well, and these need to be identified and removed from the diet.[226]

Nutrient deficiencies have been implicated in the onset and progression of OA.[209, 210] Increasing consumption of organic fruits and vegetables is a good way to increase the body's nutritional status. Since food storage and processing decreases the nutrient content of foods, patients should consume fresh, whole foods as often as possible. The saying, "eat a rainbow a day" is often useful in helping patients conceptualize what should be in their diets. Antioxidants, minerals, and other phytonutrients create the colors in fresh fruits and vegetables. Eating a variety of colorful vegetables helps ensure patients are getting a variety of healthy nutrients.

Supplements

Supplementation is an important component of OA treatment. Patients should be on a high-quality multivitamin and multimineral supplement with digestive enzymes. The best quality vitamin and mineral formulas are *not* one-a-day pills. A good supplement will be taken two to three times a day with food. And remember, these are *supplements*; they are not meant to take the place of a high quality, nutritious diet.

Evidence indicates that continuous exposure to pro-oxidants contributes to the development of many common age-related disease, including OA.[227] Dietary antioxidants include ascorbate (vitamin C) and the tocopherols (vitamin E) and beneficial effects of high doses have been reported especially in OA.[228] There is also evidence for beneficial effects of beta-carotene and selenium, the latter being a component of the antioxidant enzyme glutathione peroxidase.[228]

The following is a list of supplements were taken from Murray and Pizzorno[225] unless otherwise noted. These supplements may be of benefit for improving the symptoms and degenerative process of OA:

- Glucosamine sulfate: 1,500 mg/day
- Niacinamide: 500 mg six times/day (under strict supervision—liver enzyme must be regularly assayed)
- Vitamin E: 600 IU/day
- Vitamin A: 5,000 IU/day
- Vitamin C: 1,000–3,000 mg/day
- Vitamin B_6: 50 mg/day

- Pantothenic acid: 12.5 mg/day
- SAM: 400 mg three times/day
- Zinc: 45 mg/day
- Copper: 1 mg/day
- Boron: 6 mg/day
- MSM: 6–8 g/d. Patients may begin with two grams per day. Stiffness may not respond to this dose, but improvement may still be achieved by increasing the dose gradually (i.e., one to two additional grams each week until a clinical benefit is achieved). Treatment needs to be engaged over the long-term. With extensive involvement of the larger joints, Jacob and Appleton observed graded, dose-dependent improvememments with amounts up to 16–20 grams MSM per day.[202]
- Fish oil: 2–3 teaspoons or 3–6 capsules of high-quality fish oil per day. Fish oils are potent natural anti-inflammatories.[229, 230] Preparations can be high in vitamin A, so people at risk of vitamin A toxicity should ensure that their fish oil contains low amounts or no vitamin A. Pregnant women should consume no more than 10,000 IU vitamin A per day.
- Green lipid mussel powder (*Perna canaliculus* [Lyprinol])[231]

Topicals

- Capsaicin cream (0.025–0.05%) for pain relief. Capsaicin, which is from the cayenne pepper plant, depletes substance P. Substance P transmits pain impulses and is increased in some chronic pain conditions. Apply a thin film of capsaicin cream to the symptomatic joint four times daily. A local burning sensation is common but rarely leads to discontinuation of therapy.[232]
- Joint Comfort Cream by Herb Technology; an ointment containing thymol and other botanicals. Apply once to three times a day. Might be mildly rubefacent. Promotes circulation to the joint and increased mobility. Results may not be apparent for four to twelve weeks. Expect increased pain-free range of motion.[233]
- Traumeel homeopathic for pain relief
- MSM for pain relief and reduction of inflammation

Injectables

- Intramuscular
  - o Glucosamine: 0.5–1.0 cc each week. Combine with vitamins B12, B comp, and folate
  - o MSM
- Intra-articular
  - o MSM
  - o Superoxide disumutase (SOD)[234, 235]
  - o Traumeel homeopathic
  - o Hyaluronate
  - o Prolotherapy (12.5% to 25% dextrose) in cases of ligament laxity[236] (See Prolotherapy in the Modalities Chapter.)
- Intravenous
  - o Nutrient replacement with glucosamine added

Botanical medicines

These recommendations are from Murray and Pizzorno[225] unless otherwise noted.

- *Medicago sativa*: equivalent to 5–10 g/day
- Yucca leaves: 2–4 g three times/day
- *Harpagophytum procumbens*
  - o dried powdered root 1–2 g three times/day
  - o tincture (1:5) 4–5 ml three times/day
  - o dry solid extract (3:1) 400 mg three times/day
- *Boswellia serrata*: equivalent to 333mg boswellic acids three times/day.[237]
- *Commiphora mukul* (guggul): 500 mg three times a day with food.[238]

Homeopathy

- *Ruta graveolans*[239]

Physical therapy and exercise

Physical activity that induces physiologic or traumatic strain, such as occupational or recreational overuse of a joint, must be avoided. Normalization of posture and orthopedic correction of structural abnormalities should be utilized to limit joint strain. Short-wave diathermy, hydrotherapy, and other physical therapy modalities that improve joint perfusion are indicated.

Daily non-traumatic exercise (isometrics and swimming) is important but should be carefully monitored. Therapeutic and recreational exercises are an effective therapy in the successful management of osteoarthritis. Minor[240] reported that exercise is integral in reducing impairment, improving function, and preventing disability in OA patients. Some of the exercise benefits that accrue in this patient population are flexibility, muscular conditioning, and cardiovascular and general health.

The amount of disease progression may decrease someone's ability to participate in exercise. Range of motion exercises may help maintain joint mobility. Additionally, low-impact stretching exercises, such as gentle yoga therapy, is beneficial in many types of arthritis, including OA.[241]

Hydrotherapy

Local contrast hydrotherapy can increase circulation to a specific area of the body, flush out toxins, and increase oxygen delivery. Apply hot water to affected area for three minutes, followed by thirty seconds of ice cold water. This therapy also acts as a local analgesic and should reduce pain for several hours.

Pharmacological therapy

- Metronidozole (Flagyll): two grams on two consecutive days for six weeks. Consume *no* alcohol during this time to avoid an Antabuse (disulfiram) reaction. Gaby[226] reports 40% success with this therapy for rheumatologic conditions. Microbial die-off may cause a Herksimer reaction. To avoid this, use IM 40–80 mg depomedrol for the first week.[226]

Case: Osteoarthritis of the Knee

A fifty-four-year-old woman had suffered for years with degenerative joint disease in both of her knees. She loved to hike, ride horses, and ski but had to stop doing these activities because of the pain they would cause. She was taking Aleve, Ibuprofen, or Tylenol every day for the pain. She had been previously diagnosed with bilateral osteoarthritis. The pain was worse with physical activity and walking down stairs. She rated the pain as ten out of ten, with ten being worst, with any exertion.

After an evaluation by Dr. Neustadt, a series of prolotherapy injections were started. After a series of four injections, she was completely pain free and was able to resume her active lifestyle again. She was so thrilled with the results that she wrote the following testimonial:

"Prolotherapy was the right choice for me. My knee joint was painful, hot to the touch, and the knee cap snapped and popped. X-rays showed the joint had deteriorated significantly. After three treatments the ligaments and tendons had regained normal function and flexibility, and I was pain free.

"Prolotherapy is a proven technique that has been around since the 1930s, and I had read about it in golf magazines. Unlike cortisone, an injection that masks the pain, Prolotherapy restores joint integrity. Prolotherapy costs significantly less than orthopedic surgery and with no downtime. I had not realized that over time I had given up horseback riding, golfing, hiking, snowshoeing, and cross country skiing because it hurt. I no longer use the excuse 'I can't, I have bad knees.' I'm enjoying an active life again thanks to Dr. Neustadt and Prolotherapy."

—Joan, age fifty-four, Bozeman, MT

Chapter Eleven

Polyarthralgia

Occasionally physicians encounter patients whose symptoms do not fit neatly into a major category of disease, such as osteoarthritis, rheumatoid arthritis or psoriatic arthritis. All conventional laboratory tests are negative. There is no joint erythema, edema or calor. And physical examination does not reveal any findings. This is frequently the case with migratory polyarthralgias. However, this elusive condition may easily be explained by gut dysfunction, as discussed earlier.

Case: Severe Joint Pain in a Forty-one-year-old Man

A forty-one-year-old man complained of severe joint and muscle pains that started three years earlier. The pain was so severe that he said it felt like he his "whole body was in a pressure suit." He was unable to enjoy basic activities because of the pain. Additionally, he also suffered from insomnia, restless leg syndrome, and constipation. It would take him an hour of lying in bed to fall asleep, and his restless leg syndrome would wake him up multiple times during the night. He would only have a bowel movement every four to five days.

Dr. Pieczenik

First, this patient would have been referred to a neurologist for evaluation of the restless leg syndrome and insomnia. He may have been prescribed Mirapax or low-dose Sinemet (a medication also used for Parkinson Disease). In order to rule out any bone tumors because of the full-body "pressure" pain, he may have received a bone scan. Subsequently, if these were all negative, which they were because the patient did have a similar workup, he would have been referred to a psychologist or psychiatrist for stress management. He likely would be prescribed an anxiolytic medication such as a benzodiazepine medication for anxiety and insomnia. He also might be given an anti-inflammatory such as Vioxx. Ultimately, he would be (and in fact was) told that there was nothing else the doctors could do about it.

Dr. Neustadt

This case is a classic example from a naturopathic medical perspective of "treat the gut." This underlying cause of this patient's symptoms could be explained by underlying nutritional deficiencies such as glycine, which can cause anxiety, and severe food allergies and hyperpermeable gut, which can cause all of his symptoms. This is the Law of Parsimony. In fact, his test revealed all of these causes and the treatment plan relieved them, ultimately saving the medical system hundreds of thousands of dollars in worthless workups and treatments this patient would have suffered through the rest of his life. He in fact had already wasted tens of thousands of dollars pursuing completely fruitless evaluations and treatments prior to contacting Dr. Neustadt.

His MetaCT 400 test results revealed: (1) moderate or severe allergies to milk, casein (a protein found in high quantities in milk), eggs (white and yolk), peanuts, pistachios, mustard greens, and spinach; (2) moderately elevated cardiovascular disease risk indicated by high fibrinogen; (3) low-normal manganese; (4) exposure to aluminum and lead; (5) low vitamins A and beta-carotene; (6) elevated free radical damage to DNA (elevated 8-Hydroxy-2-deoxyguanosine); (7) vitamin D2 deficiency, putting you at increased risk for colorectal cancer; (8) low omega-3 fatty acids, which are anti-inflammatory; (9) multiple amino acid deficiencies.

Amino acid deficiencies				
Arginine	52		50 - 160	50 — 160
Histidine	78		70 - 140	70 — 140
Isoleucine	47	L	50 - 160	50 — 160
Leucine	97		90 - 200	90 — 200
Lysine	155		150 - 300	150 — 300
Methionine	24	L	25 - 50	25 — 50

Phenylalanine	44	L	45 - 140	
Threonine	152		100 - 250	
Tryptophan	28	L	35 - 65	
Valine	187		170 - 420	
Glycine	250		225 - 450	
Serine	87	L	90 - 210	
Taurine	60		50 - 250	
Tyrosine	53		50 - 120	

Mineral deficiency of manganese, which is required as an antioxidant

Manganes	32	

Deficiencies in antioxidants

Coenzyme Q10	0.54	
Vitamin A	0.50	L
ß-Carotene	0.21	L

Elevated 8-Hydroxy-2-deoxyguanosine, indicating free radical damage to DNA, a risk factor for cancer and other conditions

8-Hydroxy-2-deoxyguanosine	5.8	H

Low vitamin D

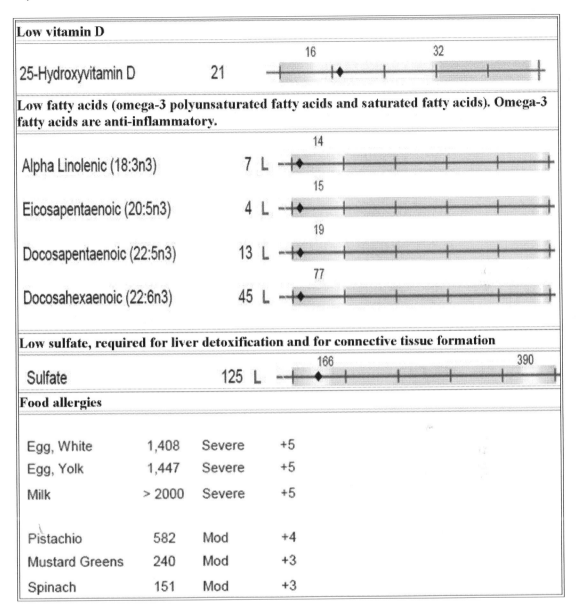

25-Hydroxyvitamin D	21	

16   32

Low fatty acids (omega-3 polyunsaturated fatty acids and saturated fatty acids). Omega-3 fatty acids are anti-inflammatory.

Alpha Linolenic (18:3n3)   7 L   14

Eicosapentaenoic (20:5n3)   4 L   15

Docosapentaenoic (22:5n3)   13 L   19

Docosahexaenoic (22:6n3)   45 L   77

Low sulfate, required for liver detoxification and for connective tissue formation

Sulfate   125 L   166   390

Food allergies

Egg, White	1,408	Severe	+5
Egg, Yolk	1,447	Severe	+5
Milk	> 2000	Severe	+5
Pistachio	582	Mod	+4
Mustard Greens	240	Mod	+3
Spinach	151	Mod	+3

He was instructed to eliminate food allergies for eight weeks while following a gut restoration program. Specific nutrients were also recommended to him as dietary supplements to correct his underlying deficiencies. After two weeks on the program, this gentleman reported that his restless leg syndrome decreased by 80%, he no longer experienced any insomnia, his muscle pain and cramps decreased by 70%, and he no longer had any constipation. At the end of his program after three months, he reported that he no longer suffered from any restless leg syndrome, brain fog, constipation, and muscle or joint pain. All of his initial complaints had completely resolved.

In an e-mail thanking NBI Testing and Consulting Corp and Dr. Neustadt, he wrote:

"You can imagine my surprise when I received the reports from my MetaCT-400 lab study and discovered I was severely allergic to dairy products, egg yolks, egg whites, and peanuts. So prior to my scheduled consultation, I immediately stopped consuming these items and foods that contained these ingredients. Three days later, I felt like a new person. Most of the chronic muscle, bone and joint aches I have been having for over ten years went away. I felt stronger, lighter on my feet, and for the first time I tired out my children while playing with them outside. The "restless leg" condition I have been having at night stopped too. The slight depression I felt was lifted as well. I now sleep better, deeper, and wake up more refreshed. I have been to sleep studies and have seen many doctors, and nothing has helped as immediately and as noticeably as the removal of these foods from my diet.

"I would have considered the food allergy results alone a complete and overwhelming success. However, the lab study also identified excessive deficiencies in my amino acids, omega fatty acids, vitamin D, essential minerals, and elevated levels of free radical damage. A replenishment program was tailored around my requirements and allergies. There is so much to learn, but Dr. Neustadt and his staff make the process simple and easy to understand. Although there are some eating and exercise habits I must change, I look forward to the many added benefit this holistic approach to health care has to offer."

—JN, Trussville, AL

Treatment Plan

Diet:

AVOID all *milk, casein (a protein found in high quantities in milk), eggs (white and yolk), peanuts, pistachios, mustard greens, and spinach* for eight weeks. See the handouts on egg allergies and alternatives to milk products.

For amino acids:

CUSTOMIZED AMINO ACID BLEND: Use as directed on the bottle.

GLYCINE POWDER: Mix ½ teaspoon daily with water with or between meals. Take one bottle of this and then discontinue.

TAURINE POWDER: Take 1/2 teaspoon daily on an empty stomach (thirty minutes before eating or 1.5 hours after eating). Take one bottle of this and then discontinue.

For vitamins and minerals:

SUPREME MULTIVITAMIN (WITHOUT IRON): Take four capsules daily with a meal.

MAG-10: Take one capsule daily with a meal.

For vitamin D:

SUPER D3: Take one capsule daily with food.

For Low Omega-3 Fatty Acids:

CARLSON'S COD LIVER OIL: Take one tablespoon (equivalent of three teaspoons) daily. Keep refrigerated.

For elevated 8-Hydroxy-2-deoxyguanosine:

VITAL MIXED ASCORBATES: Mix one scoop daily in water, and take with a meal.

To increase vitamin D:

SUPER D3, by Allergy Research Group, sixty capsules. Each capsule contains 2000 IU vitamin D3, 20 IU vitamin E, and 2 mg vitamin C. Take one capsule daily with food.

For vitamin B12:

B-12 SUBLINGUAL: Take one bottle of this and then discontinue.

To increase ability to utilize carbohydrate to create cellular energy:
MITOFORTE: Take four capsules each morning with breakfast.

COFACTOR: Take one capsule daily with food.

For low sulfur:
N-ACETYL-CYSTEINE (NAC) 1,000 mg: Take one capsule daily with food.

Case: Migratory Arthritis in a Forty-eight-year-old Woman

A forty-eight-year-old woman suffered for five years with migratory, polyarticular (multiple joints) pain throughout her body; however, the joints most affected were her knees, ankles, and hands. Her joint pain was debilitating and kept her from her favorite pastime, riding horses. She used to raise horses and at one time had thirty horses. She also complained of pain, fatigue, restlessness, depression, and being overweight. When she was first evaluated her energy was four or five out of ten (ten being best) and she reported days when her energy was zero out of ten. She slept three to four hours nightly, although she said that she would actually lie in bed for up to eight hours each night. She suffered from insomnia, with difficulty falling asleep. Her stress had been quite high, which she rated a 9.5 out of ten (ten being worst) for the four to five years prior. Her goal was to feel well enough to ride horses again. She was also overweight and unable to drop the excess pounds.

She took the MetaCT 400 test and her results revealed:

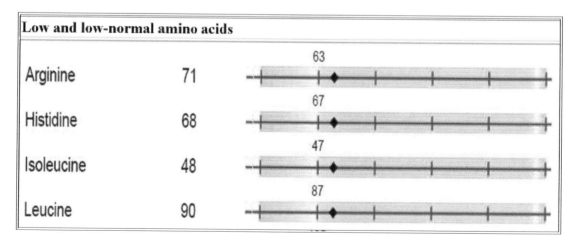

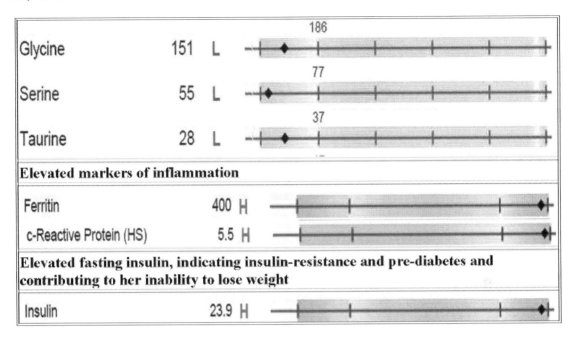

		186
Glycine	151 L	
		77
Serine	55 L	
		37
Taurine	28 L	

Elevated markers of inflammation

Ferritin	400 H
c-Reactive Protein (HS)	5.5 H

Elevated fasting insulin, indicating insulin-resistance and pre-diabetes and contributing to her inability to lose weight

Insulin	23.9 H

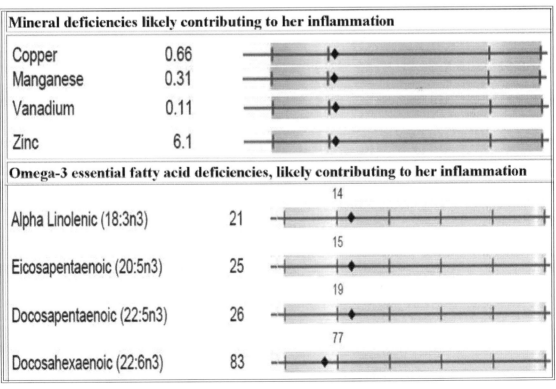

Mineral deficiencies likely contributing to her inflammation

Copper	0.66
Manganese	0.31
Vanadium	0.11
Zinc	6.1

Omega-3 essential fatty acid deficiencies, likely contributing to her inflammation

		14
Alpha Linolenic (18:3n3)	21	
		15
Eicosapentaenoic (20:5n3)	25	
		19
Docosapentaenoic (22:5n3)	26	
		77
Docosahexaenoic (22:6n3)	83	

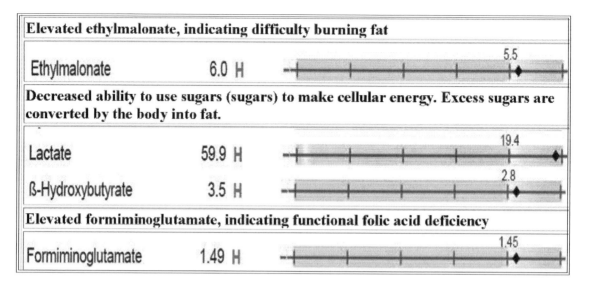

This woman was provided dietary and exercise recommendations to help her lose weight. She was referred to a physical trainer to put her on a therapeutic exercise program. She also began taking specific dietary supplements to correct her nutritional deficiencies, eliminate the infection, and improve her ability to burn her sugars and fats for energy. While on the program, her joint pain resolved, her energy increased, her food cravings for sugar were decreased, her insomnia went away, and she began to finally lose weight after years of frustrations.

Chapter Twelve

Attention Deficit Hyperactivity Disorder (ADHD)

Attention Deficit Hyperactivity Disorder (ADHD) is a condition that becomes apparent in some children in the preschool and early school years. It is hard for these children to control their behavior and/or pay attention. It is estimated that between 3 and 5% of children have ADHD, or approximately two million children in the United States. This means that in a classroom of twenty-five to thirty children, it is likely that at least one will have ADHD.

The principal characteristics of ADHD are inattention, hyperactivity, and impulsivity. These symptoms appear early in a child's life. Because many normal children may have these symptoms, but at a low level, or the symptoms may be caused by another disorder, it is important that the child receive a thorough examination and appropriate diagnosis by a well-qualified professional. The conventional approach to ADHD is to prescribe medications such as Adderrall, Concerta, Cylert, Dexedrine, Focalin, Metadate, and Ritalin.

Dr. Pieczenik

Since the DSM-I was created, psychiatry no longer became a science or art. It began to creep into "fungible diagnoses." Psychiatry, like other medical disciplines, became a field whose diagnoses and subsequent treatments, became limited to those that could be reimbursed by an insurance company.

ADHD is a good example. If clinicians label a child as having ADHD they will be reimbursed for their time and treatments. The fact that a child may be inattentive speaks to the fact that you have a characterological problem and a developmental problem. This does not mean that a child has ADHD. You may also have a problem that the environment of the child is not stimulating. It may be that the teacher is not very good or the lessons are not being taught in a way that is engaging the child's interest or the child. Unfortunately, inattention carries a very heavy loading in determining the diagnosis of ADHD. Therefore, many parents who find their children are inattentive will often resort to the highly commercialized diagnosis called ADHD. In fact, the sad truth is that neither the social context nor the person doing the observation may be qualified to make that diagnosis.

The greater problem resides in determining what is or what is not hyperactive, another diagnostic criteria for ADHD. More often than not in Dr. Pieczenik's experience, the person most qualified to tell him what the child's behavior is like is usually the mother. The problem is that the definition of hyperactivity is very subjective. One mother may have a low tolerance for activity in her child, especially in boys, who are often considered innately more restless. Therefore the mother would complain that the child is hyperactive when in fact it may just be normal behavior. Or in fact, the behavior may simply be a reaction to a family situation, such as family quarrels, or a possible depression in another family member. In this case, indeed the child may be hyperactive for very good reasons. So the context of the child's behavior as well as the observer's biases and own agenda become extremely important in the diagnosis of ADHD.

That leaves the last diagnostic criteria—impulsivity. This is a function, again, of the subjective observation as well as the developmental stage of the child. So that when you combine the three criteria together what happens is that doctors are bracketing the future of a child by giving that child medication based on behavior that may not be there in six months, one year or more. Certainly this triad of characteristics do not warrant medicating millions of children and stigmatizing their future with such a diagnosis.

And of course, no drug is without side effects. The risks in children of taking these medications include loss of appetite, increased irritability, depression, headaches, jitteriness, insomnia, increased blood pressure, suicidal behavior, psychosis, sudden death, and more. In most of Dr. Pieczenik's experience most children will grow out of two of the three diagnostic criteria. One of the precepts of medicine is, "Above all else, do no harm."

Unfortunately, in the case of ADHD, Dr. Pieczenik believes conventional medicine is doing a lot of harm to the vast majority of children who have been unnecessarily placed on these drugs. Between 1993 and 2003 ADHD medications killed nineteen children[242] and an additional twenty-six reports were recorded of strokes and rapid heart rates. Now these were recorded adverse events, the reporting of which is voluntary and therefore underestimates the risk. Irrespective of that, however, these physicians and drug companies took a nonfatal condition and made it fatal for these children.

And although the risk of sudden death is rare, it is enough of a concern that the Canadian Medical Association published recommendations in 2006 for physicians to hopefully reduce the risk of sudden cardiac death from these medications.[243] Among other recommendations, doctors are instructed to screen all patients for a family history of sudden or cardiac death before prescribing these medications. Additionally, cardiac status should be evaluated periodically in patients on long-term treatment. Drs. Neustadt and Pieczenik have never heard of doctors in the U.S. screening for these warning signs. And none of the patients Dr. Neustadt has worked with over the years with patients who had been on long-term ADHD treatments had ever had their cardiac status evaluated during treatment. Physicians are prescribing these medications without proper screening or monitoring. But more importantly, once again, doctors and drug companies have turned a nonfatal condition into a potentially fatal one.

Dr. Neustadt

The fundamental question Dr. Neustadt asks himself when a child comes into his clinic with a previous diagnosis of ADHD is, "What's the underlying cause?" This therefore requires a thorough examination of the child's home and school environments, as well as sleep patterns, exercise habits, and diet. A thorough review of systems is also conducted. This approach provides crucial clues as to how Dr. Neustadt may be able to help this child and the child's family. The key is to spend the time and develop the professional skills necessary to elicit the crucial information from the child and parent.

By this approach Dr. Neustadt was able to determine in one case that the child's underlying problem was that he was simply not getting enough sleep and that his diet was likely causing intermittent hypoglycemic crises during the day. This child was getting into fights at school and had recently been expelled. To best illustrate this case, below is the Progress Notes from the actual case with all identifying information removed. In this case you see all three characteristics of ADHD, but Dr. Neustadt did not diagnose it as such for two reasons: (1) it would be incorrect; (2) falsely labeling this child would be more damaging to him and to his parents than working to remove the underlying causes.

Progress Notes

E, a ten year-old boy, comes in today with his mother, S, with the chief complaint of "anger." E has suffered from angry outbursts since he was a young child, most recently while at his school, and he has since been kicked out of his school temporarily with the request that his family get some outside help for these angry outbursts. E and his mother both report that the outbursts are more likely to occur when E is hungry, tired, being provoked, overwhelmed, or is sick. There are eight children in his class, so class size does not appear to be an issue, according to S.

In this most recent incident, E reports that he was "tired" and "overwhelmed." While at a school outing with his class he was hit in the jaw by a ball on a racquetball court, and then later had a water bottle was pushed into his teeth by another student who E then attacked and said he wanted to "kill." Frequency of outbursts: twelve incidents since November 2005. E goes to bed at 9:00 PM and get approximately seven to eight hours of sleep per night.

EXERCISE: E exercises at school but is not involved in any team sports.

DIET RECALL: His diet consists of pasta, bread, bean and cheese burritos, jam, honey, juice, and milk (cow and goat). He likes "things with sugar." His favorite dessert is ice cream, and he craves bagels.

PHYSICAL EXAMINATION: Wt: 72lbs. Ht: 4'6". The child was alert and oriented times three and in no acute distress. He is a very friendly, sweet boy who was cooperative and expressive during the visit. E appears to generally understand that he has a problem and wishes to correct it. E does have dark circles under both eyes, which he has had for years.

IMPRESSION: 312.0 under-socialized conduct disorder, aggressive type, secondary to poor sleep habits and diet.

PLAN: I prescribed a low glycemic index diet for the patient, including 27 g of protein per day. I provided them a handout on the glycemic index and a handout on sources of protein. I prescribed a bed time of 8:30 PM instead of the current 9:00 PM so that the patient is getting adequate sleep for his age. I referred them to a counselor. This plan is based on the assumption that part of the child's major problem has to do with the fact that he is hungry and tired. The combination of the two—hunger resulting from poor blood sugar control as well as being tired—lead to an inability to process information properly and contribute to his outbursts.

* * *

At the next appointment about one month later the mother reported that her child had been compliant with the recommendations. The child's behavior problems resolved. There obviously was no need to put this child on medication.

In some cases there may in fact be other underlying causes that must be investigated. Specifically, food allergies and functional nutritional deficiencies are the actual culprits for the behavior problems, as the following case illustrates.

Case: ADHD in a Seven-year-old Boy

A seven-year-old boy was brought to Montana Integrative Medicine by his mother for an evaluation for ADHD. He had been having troubles in school, including difficulty concentrating, angry outbursts, and disruptive behaviors. He also exhibited some of these symptoms at home, would frequently complain of stomach aches, and had previously been diagnosed with ADHD. His biochemical testing revealed severe food allergies to milk and wheat, an intestinal bacterial infection, and functional deficiencies in vitamin B6 and folic acid.

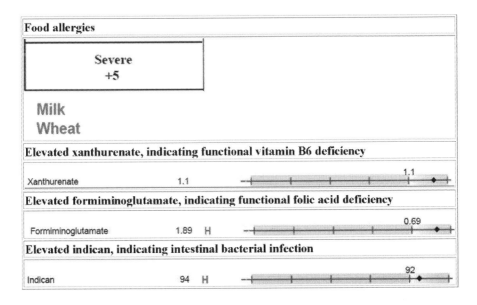

His intestinal bacterial infection was treated. He avoided milk, dairy products, and wheat. He was prescribed some dietary supplements for his deficiencies. The boy understood his behaviors were damaging, and once the results were explained to him. He agreed to comply with the recommendations. At his follow up several weeks later both he and his mother reported that all of his symptoms had improved and that he was no longer having any difficulties in school.

Treatment Plan

Diet:

AVOID all *wheat and milk products* for eight weeks, and then reintroduce them into your diet. See the handout on alternatives to milk products.

Dietary supplements:

LIQUID PEDIATRIC: Give one teaspoon with a meal once daily.

CAL/MAG: Chew two tablets once daily with a meal.

SUBLINGUAL B-6: Take ½ teaspoon daily—allow to sit under the tongue for several seconds before swallowing.

SUPER LIQUID FOLATE: Take one drop daily.

B-12 SUBLINGUAL: Dissolve one lozenge under the tongue daily.

I-FLORA 4 KIDS: Take 1/4 tsp daily water.

Case: ADHD in a Twenty-one-year-old Male

A twenty-one-year-old man contacted Dr. Neustadt for help with several complaints, chief among them being depression and attention deficit disorder, for which he had prior diagnoses and medications.

HISTORY OF PRESENT ILLNESS: The patient reports onset of depression fourteen years previously when his parents began to separate, with a subsequent divorce. He had not undergone any counseling, and he reported no history or present suicidal ideation. At the first appointment he described his mood as "apathy." His mood is better in the summer because he is partaking in more outdoor activities. The patient described difficulty concentrating, focusing on tasks, and completing tasks when not taking his Adderall. He was not exercising and because of chronic back pain.

ENERGY was seven to eight out of ten, with ten being best, while taking the Adderall, and three to four out of ten without the medication. His *sleep* was not restful. He sleeps seven to eight hours nightly, and it occasionally takes him two hours to fall asleep. He awakes after approximately two hours of sleeping secondary to back pain, and he awakes unrefreshed in the morning. The patient reported a rather high level of *stress* during the past two months secondary to difficulties in his relationship with his girlfriend. He rated his stress at eight and a half or nine out of ten, with ten being worst.

CURRENT MEDICATIONS AND DIETARY SUPPLEMENTS: Adderall XR 15 mg qd since 10/11/06. Zoldipem 10 mg qd for sleep since 11/9/07. No dietary supplements.

SOCIAL HISTORY: He had two siblings and is the middle child. He was a college student studying film, and works in retail sales fifteen hours per week. He enjoys photography, which helps him reduce his stress.

REVIEW OF SYSTEMS: General—The patient experienced headaches daily between the hours of 5:00 PM and 10:00 PM, which were self-limiting and ameliorated with drinking water. No fevers. No rashes. No weight changes. He experienced post-nasal drip two to three times weekly, with dysphagia occurring only when he has the post-nasal drip. Cardiovascular—He had been experiencing palpitations more than twice weekly secondary to stress, according to his report. No chest pain. He is having shortness of breath three to four times each week while at rest, in a sitting position, and experiences orthostatic hypotension once weekly. Gastrointestinal—No abdominal discomfort. He has one bowel movement daily without any gross hematochezia or mucous. Genitourinary—Urine appears OK—no urgency, polyuria, dysuria, or incomplete voiding. Musculoskeletal—He reports upper-, low-, and mid-back pain, which began after his second motor vehicle accident. The pain is constant and without radiation. It is slightly ameliorated with physical therapy. The pain is of a sharp quality and the intensity is about a nine out of ten, with ten being worst.

DIET RECALL: The patient does not drink coffee. Breakfast—oatmeal, water; Lunch—Soup (broccoli, chicken), water; Dinner—Pasta with shrimp, Caesar salad, sstrawberry shortcake; Cravings—chicken; Water—three glassed daily.

PHYSICAL EXAMINATION: General—The patient is alert and oriented time three and in no acute distress. Height: 67.5". Weight: 161 pounds. Temperature: 98.8 F. BP: 114/80. Pulse: 84 BPM and regular. His affect appeared flat, but he was interactive and appropriate during the interview. He was friendly and frequently elaborated on the details of his symptoms without further questioning by Dr. Neustasdt. Neurological—Achilles and patellar deep tendon reflexes are +2 bilaterally. Achilles reflexes bilaterally are without relaxation phase delay. CN 3 through 7, 11, and 12 are grossly intact.

IMPRESSION / PLAN: The patient is a pleasant, intelligent young man. He comes in with a past diagnosis of Attention Deficit Disorder (ADD) and depression. I discussed with him the possible underlying metabolic causes of ADD and depression, and recommended a MetaCT 150 test to evaluate him for fasting plasma amino acids, urinary organic acids, and food allergies. I spoke to him about getting some counseling for the depression, which he'd never gotten in the past. He declined my offer to refer him to a local counselor. I also ordered a Met-C, CBC with differential, and TSH tests through a local lab. I also provided approximately fifteen minutes of nutritional counseling and calculated his U.S. RDA for protein and provided specific recommendations for protein and fruits/vegetables.

* * *

His MetaCT 150 test results revealed:

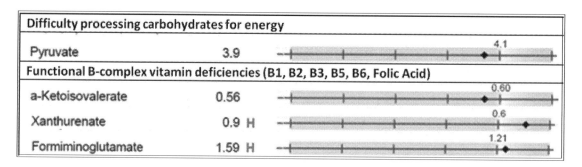

Decreased markers for norepinephrine, epinephrine and Homovanillate		
Vanilmandelate	1.8	1.1 ——◆—— 3.8
Homovanillate	< 0.1 L	1.6 ◆—— 7.7
Elevated marker of free radical damage		
p-Hydroxyphenyllactate	1.4 H	0.7 ——◆
Decreased sulfur		
Sulfate	54 L	123 ◆—— 343
Amino acid deficiencies		
Methionine	17	17 ——◆——
Valine	152 L	159 ◆——
Serine	65 L	66 ◆——
Taurine	26 L	36 ◆——
Tyrosine	41 L	43 ◆——

Treatment Plan

For ability to better utilize sugars for cellular energy:
MITOFORTE: Take four capsules each morning with breakfast.

COFACTOR B: Take one capsule daily with food.

FA-8 FOLIC ACID: Take one capsule daily. Take one bottle and then discontinue.

MAG-10: Take one capsule daily with a meal.

AN-30: Take one capsule twice daily with a meal.

SAMe, 200 mg: Take one or two tablets daily.

For amino acids:
RESCULPT: Stir or blend two scoops (23g) of ReSculpt into 8 fl. oz. of water, milk, or juice once daily.

TAURINE POWDER: Take 1/2 teaspoon daily. Take one bottle of this and then discontinue.

TYROSINE 1g: Take one table daily.

For liver detoxification pathways:
N-ACETYL-CYSTEINE (NAC) 900 mg: Take one capsule daily with food.

For antioxidants:
BUFFERED VITAMIN C 1,000 mg: Take two capsules daily.

CURCUMIN PRO: Take one tablet twice daily.

* * *

After three months on the treatment plan the patient reported that this approach had "stabilized things." He had completely discontinued his Adderall and Zoldipem medications without any difficulties or adverse effects. His energy without the Adderall was eight to nine out of ten, according to the patient, with ten being best. Prior to the treatment plan his energy without the Adderall was three to four out of ten, with ten being best. He could focus mentally for far longer periods than before and complete tasks without difficulties. His depression resolved completely, and he no longer experienced mood fluctuations. His sleep was "good," his post-nasal drip had resolved, as did his palpitations. The patient stated unequivocally that the treatment plan based on the testing was a "complete success."

In this patient follow-up amino acid and urinary organic acids testing was done, which showed significant positive changes in all variables, which corresponded to his clinical improvement.

Chapter Thirteen

Depression

The underlying pathophysiology of major depressive disorder (MDD) has not been clearly defined. Clinical and preclinical trials suggest a disturbance in CNS serotonin (i.e., 5-HT) activity as an important factor. Other neurotransmitters implicated include norepinephrine (NE) and dopamine (DA).

The role of CNS serotonin activity in the pathophysiology of MDD is suggested by the efficacy of selective serotonin reuptake inhibitors (SSRIs) in the treatment of MDD. Furthermore, studies have shown that an acute, transient relapse of depressive symptoms can be produced in research subjects in remission using tryptophan depletion, which causes a temporary reduction in CNS serotonin levels. Serotonergic neurons implicated in affective disorders are found in the dorsal raphe nucleus, the limbic system, and the left prefrontal cortex.

Clinical experience indicates a complex interaction between neurotransmitter availability, receptor regulation and sensitivity, and affective symptoms in MDD. Drugs that produce only an acute rise in neurotransmitter availability, such as cocaine, do not have efficacy over time as antidepressants. Furthermore, an exposure of several weeks' duration to an antidepressant usually is necessary to produce a change in symptoms. This, together with preclinical research findings, implies a role for neuronal receptor regulation over time in response to enhanced neurotransmitter availability.

All available antidepressants appear to work via one or more of the following mechanisms:

(1) presynaptic inhibition of uptake of 5-HT or NE; (2) antagonist activity at presynaptic inhibitory 5-HT or NE receptor sites, thereby enhancing neurotransmitter release; or (3) inhibition of monoamine oxidase, thereby reducing neurotransmitter breakdown.

Depression is a clinical diagnosis, meaning lab tests are not used to identify depression. Symptoms vary from person to person and causes changes in thinking, feeling, behavior, and physical well-being, including difficulty concentrating and making decisions, forgetfulness, negative thoughts (e.g., pessimism, poor self-esteem, excessive guilt, self-criticism), self-destructive thoughts, sadness, loss of enjoyment or interest in activities, decreased motivation, apathy, lethargy, irritability, decreased libido, fatigue, and insomnia.

People with many other conditions may also be suffering from depression. Many cases of depression have been evaluated and effectively improved with this nutritional biochemical approach. Dr. Neustadt has charted more than 95% success rate, defined as as 80% or greater reduction of depression symptoms, treating depression in his clinic with his approach to biochemical testing and treatments. Other conditions with depression as a major component include arthritis, seizure disorder, irritable bowel syndrome (IBS), Lyme disease, migraine headaches, and multiple sclerosis.

Dr. Pieczenik

Depression manifests itself in many different ways, such as anxiety, insomnia, psychosomatic complaints, inability to work or have fun, and of course, suicide. Depression entails both a biological and a cultural component. The biological component clearly has genetic determinants, termed "endogenous depression." In this particular case one would expect to have some form of depression or its manifestation throughout one's life. This is much harder to treat than its converse, reactive depression. This occurs in situations where there is a lot of stress, such as death of a loved one, divorce, loss of a job, and financial bankruptcy. Many addictions and other psychiatric diagnoses really mask an underlying depression. In many cases the solution to a depression is either to drink it away or to engage in promiscuous and high-risk activities. These all result in a form of self-destructive behavior in the goal of trying to terminate one's life without it being labeled "suicide."

In both endogenous and reactive depression the antidepressants, whether the MAO inhibitors, SSRIs, Tricylic antidepressants, atypical antidepressants, lithium, or anticonvulsants, are largely ineffectual.

As already mentioned in the foreword to this book, the NEJM reported in 2008 that the effectiveness of antidepressant medications had been overstated by as much as 61% by the suppression of negative studies by the pharmaceutical industries and the FDA.[82] An alternative approach is required in order to understand the underlying biochemical analytes that contribute to the affective disorders.

Dr. Neustadt

Depression is one of the most common complaints I hear in my clinic. The biochemical pathways for depression and energy production are well documented. Without being too complicated, the mood-lifting hormone serotonin is produced in the body by transforming the amino acid tryptophan into serotonin, and requires vitamin B6 and magnesium to do so. Other biochemical deficiencies that are associated with depression are iron deficiency, hypothyroidism, vitamin B12 deficiency, folic acid deficiency, and more. In addition to identifying and treating the underlying biochemical causes of this condition, frequently referral to a counselor is helpful, as is ensuring patients are eating an optimal diet and getting adequate exercise and sleep.

Case: Depression in a Thirty-five-year-old Woman

A thirty-five-year-old woman came to Dr. Neustadt after suffering from life-long depression. She was unable to work because of her depression and had been taking 20 mg of Lexapro daily for the previous two years. Despite the medication and seeing a counselor, her depression was worsening. She also complained of abdominal gas and bloating, mood swings, anxiety, fatigue, apathy, irritability, poor concentration, and difficulty making decisions. She had no history of suicide attempts.

Her MetaCT 400 test results revealed:

Low essential amino acids, which can cause poor blood sugar control		
Isoleucine	43	L
Leucine	86	L
Lysine	159	
Methionine	27	
Phenylalanine	41	L
Threonine	104	
Tryptophan	39	
Valine	181	

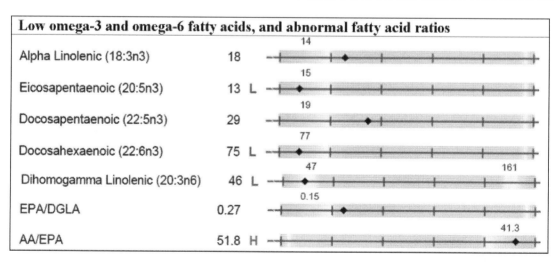

Low erythrocyte minerals

Chromium	0.24	L
Copper	0.45	L
Magnesium	30	L
Manganese	0.28	
Potassium	1,350	
Selenium	0.14	
Vanadium	0.10	
Zinc	4.8	L

Low CoQ10

Coenzyme Q10	0.53

Vitamin A	0.50	L
ß-Carotene	0.71	

Elevated markers of free radical damage

8-Hydroxy-2-deoxyguanosine	5.5	H
p-Hydroxyphenyllactate	2.4	H

Low vitamin D

25-hydroxyvitamin D	L	12

Low omega-3 and omega-6 fatty acids, and abnormal fatty acid ratios

Alpha Linolenic (18:3n3)	18	
Eicosapentaenoic (20:5n3)	13	L
Docosapentaenoic (22:5n3)	29	
Docosahexaenoic (22:6n3)	75	L
Dihomogamma Linolenic (20:3n6)	46	L
EPA/DGLA	0.27	
AA/EPA	51.8	H

Elevated pyruvate, indicating decreased ability to burn sugars for energy			
Pyruvate	4.4 H		4.1
a-Ketoglutarate	102.0 H		38.7
Succinate	15.9		18.3
Functional B-complex (B1, B2, B3, B5 and B6) vitamins			
a-Ketoisocaproate	0.39		0.39
Xanthurenate	0.7		0.8
Moderate and severe food allergies			
Casein	1,243	Severe	+5
Milk	292	Mod	+3
Navy Bean	164	Mod	+3
Ginger	> 2000	Severe	+5
Almond	171	Mod	+3

Over the course of the three-month treatment plan, the patient's condition markedly improved. She was able to discontinue her Lexapro, her abdominal discomforts resolved, her energy improved, as did her tendency toward irritability and angry outbursts. Overall she reported that she felt much better and more decisive. She was able to resume working and even returned to college for a degree in nursing. Her depression did not completely resolve, and she ended up getting back on an antidepressant medication—Welbutrin. However, what this case demonstrates is that improvement occurred to the point where a woman who was completely debilitated and unable to participate in life was subsequently able to feel better and start a career.

* * *

Treatment Plan

Diet:
AVOID all *casein (a protein that's high in dairy products), dairy, all dairy products, navy beans, ginger, and almonds* for eight weeks, and then reintroduce them into your diet. See the handout on alternatives to milk products.

Dietary supplements:
SUPREME FEM MULTIVITAMIN (WITH IRON): Take four capsules daily with a meal.

MITOFORTE: Take two capsules each morning with breakfast.

COFACTOR B: Take one capsule daily with food.

MAG-10: Take one capsule daily with a meal.

EMERGEN-C PACKETS: Take two packets three times daily, if tolerated.

CARLSON'S COD LIVER OIL: Take one tablespoon (equivalent of three teaspoons) daily.

EVENING PRIMROSE OIL: Take two soft gels twice daily or four soft gels once daily with a meal.

VITAMIN D3, 5,000 IU: Take one capsule daily with food.

GLUTAMINE RX: Mix one teaspoon twice daily in water and drink.

PROMINERALS: Take three capsules daily with food. Take two bottles and then discontinue.

ULTRA PROTEIN PLUS - CHOCOLATE ALMOND POWDER: Mix one heaping scoop daily in a liquid of your choice.

TAURINE POWDER: Take 1/2 teaspoon daily on an empty stomach (thirty minutes before eating or 1.5 hours *after eating). Take one bottle and then discontinue.*

ENTEROPRO: Take one capsule daily with food. Keep refrigerated.

Case: Depression in a Twenty-three-year-old Man

A twenty-three-year-old man came to see Dr. Neustadt complaining of suffering from depression. He would sleep ten to twelve hours daily and would wake up repeatedly during the night. His energy was five out of ten, with ten being best, which he characterized as "low." He had been experiencing this low energy level for five years. He did not exercise, and his stress was nine out of ten with ten being worst, secondary to "government and world issues." He had been divorced and had partial custody of his three-year-old son. When asked about his mood, he replied, "I hate people." His affect was flat during the first appointment, although he was very honest and forthcoming with his emotions and in discussing his feelings. He had no history of suicidal ideation or attempts.

He took the MetaCT 150 test, which revealed:

Decreased hormone markers for norepinephrine/epinephrine (Vanilmandelate), dopamine (Homovanillate) and serotonin (5-Hydroxyindoleacetate)		
Vanilmandelate	1.5	1.1 — 3.8
Homovanillate	1.4 L	1.6 — 7.7
5-Hydroxyindoleacetate	1.7	1.5 — 6.3
Decreased amino acids involved in hormone production (phenylalanine and tyrosine for the production of dopamine and norepinephrine/epinephrine and tryptophan for the production of serotonin)		
Phenylalanine	48	48
Tryptophan	35 L	38
Tyrosine	43	43
Food allergies		
Egg, White	> 2000 Severe	+5
Egg, Yolk	1,817 Severe	+5

During the treatment plan, his depression completely resolved, and his energy increased. After six weeks on the plan, he characterized his mood as "happy." He also reported that he had no more stress, his sleep was "good," and he did not wake up during the night anymore. Additionally, his energy had increased to eight out of ten, with ten being best. He mentioned after twelve weeks on the program that the few times that he did not comply with the dietary recommendations on the treatment plan that he felt a return of his symptoms.

* * *

Treatment Plan

Diet:

AVOID all *eggs and egg-containing products* for eight weeks, then reintroduce them into your diet. See the handout on egg allergies.

For amino acids:

RESCULPT: Stir or blend two (2) scoops (23g) of ReSculpt into 8 fl. oz. of water, milk, or juice once daily.

L-TRYPTOPHAN 500 mg: Take one capsule three times daily. Take for sixty days and then discontinue.

TYROSINE 1g: Take one table daily. Take one bottle and then discontinue.

For vitamins and minerals:

SUPREME MULTIVITAMIN (WITHOUT IRON): Take four capsules daily with a meal.

REJUVAMAG: Take one capsule each night before bed. Take one bottle and then discontinue.

PROMINERALS: Take three capsules daily with food. Take one bottle and then discontinue.

COFACTOR B: Take one capsule daily with food.

For ability to burn fats and sugars for energy:
MITOFORTE: Take four capsules each morning with breakfast.

For gut repair:
GLUTAMINE RX: Mix one teaspoon twice daily in water and drink.

For liver detoxification pathway:
N-ACETYL-CYSTEINE (NAC): Take one capsule daily with food. Take one bottle and then discontinue.

For fatty acids:
CARLSON'S COD LIVER OIL: Take one tablespoon (equivalent of three teaspoons) daily. Keep refrigerated.

Case: Endogenous Depression in a Fifty-two-year-old Woman

A fifty-two-year-old woman presented to Dr. Neustadt's clinic, Montana Integrative Medicine, with a life-long history of depression. She had suicidal thoughts as young as five years old, and attempted suicide once in the past. She also experienced insomnia and occasional migraine headaches. Her biochemical testing revealed functional deficiencies in nutrients required to generate energy and lift mood. She also complained of difficulty losing weight.

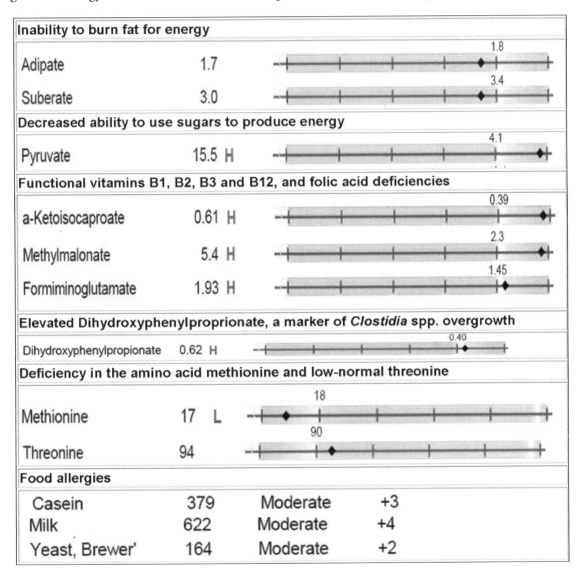

She was instructed to avoid the foods to which she was allergic, provided specific dietary recommendations, and given dietary supplements to give her body the nutrients it was lacking. Two weeks later, at her first follow-up appointment, she reported that she was following the treatment plan diligently, that her mood was "shockingly stable," and that she was not experiencing much depression or anxiety at all. After six weeks on the program, she reported continued improvement in her depression and that her pants fit looser on her. After three months, she reported complete resolution of her depression for the first time in her life.

* * *

Treatment Plan

This treatment plan is based on your interview with Dr. Neustadt; physical examination; and your MetaCT 150 test results. Your laboratory results indicate: (1) multiple functional vitamin deficiencies, (2) high stress, (3) exposure to toxic compounds, (4) intestinal bacterial dysbiosis with *Clostridia* spp., (5) several food intolerances. Each of these is shown as categories on your test report, a copy of which was provided to you. This treatment plan attempts to address these and improve your health.

Diet:
AVOID *casein, dairy, codfish, oyster, vanilla, baker's yeast, brewer's yeast, almond, mustard greens, and tomato* for eight weeks, then reintroduce them into your diet.

Stress reduction:
RELAXATION: I encourage you to do something every day for yourself to nourish your soul. Some suggestions are yoga, breathing exercises, meditation, reading, and walking. Find something that works for you, and do this regularly.

EXERCISE: This will reduce your stress. Do aerobic exercise at least three days a week for twenty minutes each time.

You may want to try "five-second breathing."

> Breathing—"five-second cycle breathing," as demonstrated in your appointment. Breathe in through the nose (deep, belly breaths) for five seconds, hold your breath for five seconds, and then breathe out through the mouth for five seconds. Repeat three, five, or more times, until you get into a calm space. Do this several times a day or as frequently as you need.

Dietary supplements

SUPREME FEM MULTIVITAMIN (WITH IRON): Take four capsules daily with a meal.

L-METHIONINE 500 mg: Take one capsule daily.

GLYCINE POWDER: Mix ½ teaspoon daily with water with or between meals.

COFACTOR B: Take one capsule daily with food.

MITOFORTE: Take four capsules each morning with breakfast.

COENZYME Q-10: Take one capsule daily with food.

B-12 SUBLINGUAL: Dissolve one lozenge under the tongue daily.

For the bacterial dysbiosis:

BERBERINE FORTE: Take one capsule twice daily with food.

ENTEROPRO: Take one capsule daily with food.

Case: Depression in a Twenty-six-year-old Woman

A twenty-six-year-old woman presented with a three-year history of depression and fatigue. She also complained that colds would linger longer for her than in others, and that she had post-nasal drip "almost all the time," pre-menstrual migraine headaches for the past eight years, abdominal gas/bloating, brain fog, orthostatic hypotension (getting light-headed when she stood up) "all the time," and an increase in ten pounds of weight in the past couple of years, which she could not lose despite how much she exercised. She rated her energy at three out of ten, with ten being best.

Her MetaCT 400 test results revealed (1) deficiencies in all ten essential amino acids; (2) iron deficiency (low ferritin); (3) multiple mineral deficiencies; (4) elevated free radical damage to cell membranes (elevated lipid peroxides); (5) low vitamin D (risk factor for breast cancer); (6) low omega-6 series fatty acids; (7) functional vitamin deficiencies for energy production; (8) impaired liver detoxification pathways; (9) intestinal bacterial and fungal overgrowth; (10) and severe food intolerances to milk, casein (a protein in milk), and eggs (white and yolk), as well as moderate intolerance to ginger.

Food allergies to dairy, eggs and ginger

Casein	> 2000	Severe	+5
Egg, White	> 2000	Severe	+5
Egg, Yolk	337	Mod	+3
Milk	> 2000	Severe	+5
Ginger	178	Mod	+3

Amino acid deficiencies

Arginine	49	L	50 - 160	50 · · · 160
Histidine	68	L	70 - 140	70 · · · 140
Isoleucine	45	L	50 - 160	50 · · · 160
Leucine	82	L	90 - 200	90 · · · 200
Lysine	145	L	150 - 300	150 · · · 300
Methionine	23	L	25 - 50	25 · · · 50
Phenylalanine	52		45 - 140	45 · · · 140
Threonine	93	L	100 - 250	100 · · · 250
Tryptophan	32	L	35 - 65	35 · · · 65
Valine	159	L	170 - 420	170 · · · 420
Tyrosine	43	L	50 - 120	50 · · · 120

Low minerals

Chromium	0.28	
Copper	0.59	
Magnesium	43	
Manganese	0.28	
Potassium	1,637	
Selenium	0.16	

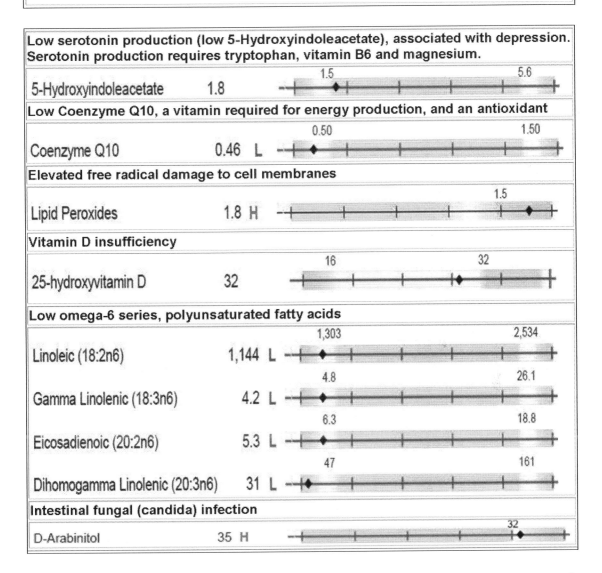

| Vanadium | 0.09 L | |
| Zinc | 6.2 | |

Low serotonin production (low 5-Hydroxyindoleacetate), associated with depression. Serotonin production requires tryptophan, vitamin B6 and magnesium.

| 5-Hydroxyindoleacetate | 1.8 | |

Low Coenzyme Q10, a vitamin required for energy production, and an antioxidant

| Coenzyme Q10 | 0.46 L | |

Elevated free radical damage to cell membranes

| Lipid Peroxides | 1.8 H | |

Vitamin D insufficiency

| 25-hydroxyvitamin D | 32 | |

Low omega-6 series, polyunsaturated fatty acids

Linoleic (18:2n6)	1,144 L	
Gamma Linolenic (18:3n6)	4.2 L	
Eicosadienoic (20:2n6)	5.3 L	
Dihomogamma Linolenic (20:3n6)	31 L	

Intestinal fungal (candida) infection

| D-Arabinitol | 35 H | |

This woman was placed on a comprehensive nutritional medicine program consisting of a combination of diet and nutraceuticals, and it was recommended that she receive counseling. After two weeks on the program she reported that her energy had already increased and that she no longer experienced post-nasal drip. After six weeks on the program she reported that her energy had increased to nine out of ten, with ten being best. She had no post-nasal drip, no migraine headaches, and no abdominal bloating, and she no longer got lightheaded when she stood up (orthostatic hypotension). Her depression had also completely resolved.

* * *

Treatment Plan

Diet:
AVOID all *milk, casein (read labels carefully), all milk products, all eggs (read labels carefully), and ginger* for eight weeks, then reintroduce them into your diet.

For intestinal fungal overgrowth:
Rx NYSTATIN TABLETS, 500,000 units twice daily for three months.

For intestinal bacterial overgrowth:
BERBERINE FORTE: Take one capsule twice daily with food.

ENTEROPRO: Take one capsule daily with food.

For amino acid deficiencies:
CUSTOMIZED AMINO ACID BLEND: Take as directed on the bottle.

GLUTAMINE RX: Mix 1 teaspoon twice daily in water and drink.

MITOFORTE: Take four capsules each morning with breakfast.

For vitamin and functional mineral deficiencies, and free radical damage:
SUPREME FEM MULTIVITAMIN (WITH IRON): Take four capsules daily with a meal.

COFACTOR B: Take one capsule daily with food.

MAG-10: Take one capsule daily with a meal.

FERROSOLVE: Take one capsule daily with or without food.

PROMINERALS: Take three capsules daily with food. Take one bottle and then discontinue.

For low omega-6 fatty acids:

EVENING PRIMROSE OIL: Take two soft gels twice daily or four soft gels once daily with a meal.

For low liver detoxification pathways:

N-ACETYL-CYSTEINE (NAC) 1000 mg: Take one capsule daily with food.

Chapter Fourteen

Narcolepsy

Narcolepsy affects 0.03-0.1% of the general population, with the onset around adolescence and with boys and girls being equally affected.[244] However, certain populations have higher prevalences of this condition: Japanese general population, 0.18%; French Caucasians, 0.05%; United Kingdom Caucasians, 0.04%; Finnish Caucasians, 0.026%; Czech Caucasians, 0.02%; and Israeli Jews and Arabs, 0.002%.

This debilitating condition is characterized by a tetrad of symptoms: (1) excessive daytime sleepiness, (2) cataplexy, (3) sleep paralysis and (4) hypnagogic hallucinations.[245-250] Hypersomnolence is such a characteristic symptom of this condition that the term "narcolepsy" in fact is derived from Greek, "seized by somnolence." Cataplexy is sudden muscle atonia in response to emotional arousal, in particular laughter. Hypnagogic hallucinations are dream-like episodes when going to sleep.

Thus, patients with narcolepsy demonstrate two major abnormalities: inability to stay awake in the daytime and REM sleep interruptions leading to wakefulness or non-restorative sleep. An overnight polysomnogram followed by a multiple sleep latency test (MSLT) is essential in the workup. The MSLT is administered during the day to assess daytime sleepiness and to diagnose narcolepsy. It consists of four or five opportunities to take 15- to 20-minute naps, each separated by a two-hour interval.[251]

In the late 1800s a familial tendency towards narcolepsy was first documented. First-degree relatives had a one to two percent risk of developing narcolepsy, which is 20-40 times higher than the general population.[244]

There is no known cause of primary narcolepsy. However, primary narcolepsy is thought to result from genetic predisposition, abnormal neurotransmitter functioning and sensitivity, and abnormal immune modulation. Secondary narcolepsy can be caused by head trauma, encephalopathy, brain tumors and cerebrovascular insufficiency.

In addition to the physically incapacitating effects of narcolepsy, this condition is also emotionally and socially awkward. Patients often feel embarrassed about their symptoms and can experience social isolation. They may not be able to drive, hold down a job or keep up with school work. In one study, 24% of narcoleptic patients had to quit working and 18% were terminated from their jobs because of their disease.

Dr. Pieczenik

Dr. Pieczenik has had only one experience with a person with narcolepsy, when he was working with the Director of the Central Intelligence Agency (DCIA), William J. Casey. At that time, Dr. Pieczenik was the Deputy Assistant Secretary of State (DAS) under President Reagan. Mr. Casey was talking over a period of several hours to Dr. Pieczenik about the Lebanese Civil War in the 1980s, and Mr. Casey would repeatedly close his eyes and nod off. While in mid-sentence Mr. Casey's voice would trail off, he would stop talking and literally fall asleep. Dr. Pieczenik and others in the room, who included some of the most famous intelligence operatives portrayed in the movies *Syriana* and *Charlie Wilson's War*, had to simply sit and wait for Mr. Casey to wake up.

Dr. Pieczenik began speaking loudly and in a brusk voice, assuming that Mr. Casey was simply tired and bored. Dr. Pieczenik had no idea that he was witnessing a real neurological phenomenon, despite the fact that he was a board examiner in neurology. This just goes to show how rare this condition is. Most clinicians never see or treat narcolepsy their entire careers. And the possibility that the director of the CIA had narcolepsy didn't even enter into Dr. Pieczenik's mind. He was incredulous. None of the operatives in the room, who knew Mr. Casey suffered from this condition, said anything about it. They all just sat quietly and waited. No matter how loud Dr. Pieczenik spoke, Mr. Casey would not wake up. Mr. Casey would drift in and out of sleep over the course of the hour-and-a-half meeting. Only months later did Dr. Pieczenik learn that Mr. Casey had narcolepsy.

There is a certain irony to the story: that no matter how educated you may be, or how sensitive the subject matters might be, the overwhelming urge to sleep in people with narcolepsy cannot be overcome. And more importantly, the fact that no one told Dr. Pieczenik, a board examiner in neurology, likely meant that Mr. Casey and his subordinates were embarrassed and uncomfortable with this condition.

Dr. Neustadt

The fact that naturopathic physicians frequently see patients who have not gotten relief from their condition by conventional means, results in many naturopathic doctors evaluating and treating conditions that the general MD family physician would not see. Fortunately, Dr. Neustadt had the occasion to help one young man with narcolepsy.

The approach in working up this case was similar to other cases—see if the underlying biochemical abnormalities could be determined and work to correct them using Targeted Nutrient Therapy™. The patient came to Dr. Neustadt via a referral from a local nutritionist.

Case: Narcolepsy in a Twenty-five-year-old Man

A twenty-five-year-old man, who had been diagnosed years earlier with narcolepsy, lived in Arizona, where he was finding it impossible to continue to work or attend school. He would literally sleep all day and all night for days at a time. In fact, he made the comment that he would "have a two hour nap before going to sleep." He had lost weight and was completely unmotivated and depressed. He rated his energy at a zero out of ten, with ten being best. He was unable to read more than a paragraph at any one time in a book. He simply could not focus his mind and he would begin to fall asleep. He was completely socially isolated.

By the time his mother found Dr. Neustadt to help her son, the family was literally exasperated and didn't know what to do. The son did not want to move home with his parents, but if his health did not improve, he would have had no other option.

This young man had been prescribed a series of different medications over the years to treat symptoms. The most recent of those was Ritalin. This amphetamine would make him feel "jittery" and "wired" but, paradoxically, he did not experience any increase in energy. On the contrary, he merely experienced an increase in anxiety and a decreased ability to focus.

His MetaCT 400 test results revealed:

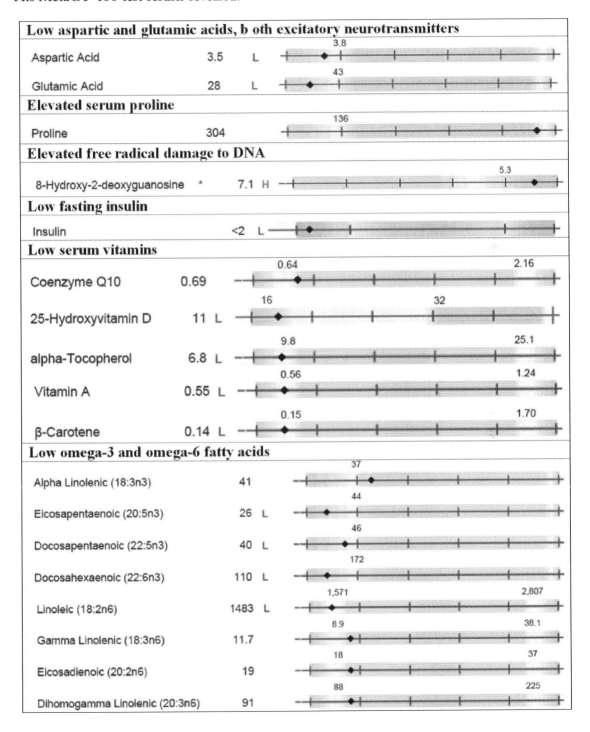

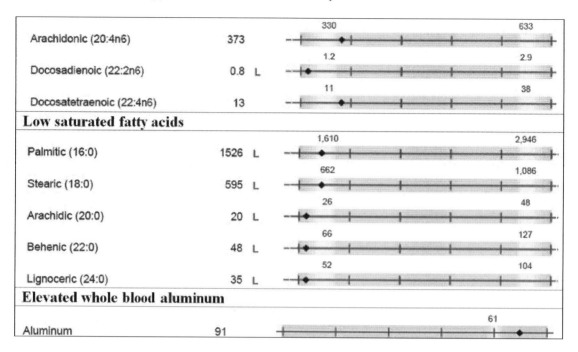

Arachidonic (20:4n6)	373		330 — 633
Docosadienoic (22:2n6)	0.8 L		1.2 — 2.9
Docosatetraenoic (22:4n6)	13		11 — 38
Low saturated fatty acids			
Palmitic (16:0)	1526 L		1,610 — 2,946
Stearic (18:0)	595 L		662 — 1,086
Arachidic (20:0)	20 L		26 — 48
Behenic (22:0)	48 L		66 — 127
Lignoceric (24:0)	35 L		52 — 104
Elevated whole blood aluminum			
Aluminum	91		61

Interestingly, Dr. Neustadt was quite surprised to learn that this patient's essential amino acids and markers for functional vitamin B deficiencies and mitochondrial dysfunction were all normal.

In researching the case to create the treatment plan, Dr. Neustadt discovered that low aspartic and glutamic acids have been associated with narcolepsy.

Aspartic acid is a precursor to oxaloacetate, a Kreb's Cycle intermediate, which is required for mitochondrial ATP production. Additionally, aspartic acid is a preferred substrate for the refilling pathway that restores Kreb's Cycle levels of citrate and isocitrate, and can help to increase these energy producing intermediates. Aspartic acid is also involved in glucose synthesis, the urea cycle and a precursor of both DNA and RNA. Low levels of aspartic acid may reflect lowered cellular energy-generating capacity, experienced as chronic fatigue.[252] In a pharmacokinetic rat study published in 1982, the simultaneous administration of aspartic acid and arginine led to increases in neurostimulatory amino acids in the brain.[253]

In 1935 none other than Hans Krebs himself, published a paper showing how proline can be converted to glutamic acid in the kidneys.[254] The oxidation of proline to glutamic acid requires niacin as a cofactor.[252] In this narcolepsy case, the man's proline was elevated, functional markers for niacin were normal (alpha-Ketoisovalerate, alpha-Ketoisocaproate and alpha-Keto-beta-Methylvalerate) and his glutamic acid was low. This could be interepreted that he has difficulty converting proline to glutamic acid. The cause may be genetic and he may require long-term glutamic acid replacement therapy. However, one caveat is important to note here. Glutamic acid when too high is a neurotoxin. Therefore, this patient may require titration of glutamic acid to achieve maximal clinical results.

Glutamic acid is involved in glucose synthesis, the urea cycle, glutathione synthesis and is a neurotransmitter. In fact, in the central nervous system (CNS), glutamic acid is *the* major excitatory neurotransmitter.[252]

Dr. Pieczenik posits that, since destruction of dopaminergic neurons by glutamic acid is an etiological factor in Parkinson's disease (PD), that narcolepsy may be viewed as the converse of PD. Therefore, Dr. Pieczenik believes that narcolepsy and PD may eventually be viewed on a spectrum of disease states associated with glutamate levels. He also speculates that schizophrenia, epilepsy and bipolar disorder are all affected by the glutaminergic system. Additional research is obviously required to investigate these hypotheses.

After being on the plan (below) for one month, the patient had a follow-up with Dr. Neustadt. At that time the patient reported that his energy had increased to 6.5 out of ten, with ten being best. He was more alert, focused and had more mental and physical stamina. He was still sleeping more than was normal, from eight o'clock at night to about noon the next day, but when he was awake he functioned normally. He was awake for eight hours a day, compared to sleeping for days in a row before the program. He was even able read multiple chapters in books at a time without falling asleep.

This case is interesting for many reasons. While the clinical results showed improvement, Dr. Neustadt is not entirely sure why. Which agent or combination of agents prescribed created the improvement? Some may view this as a limitation of this approach in medicine; however, Drs. Neustadt and Pieczenik do not agree. The substances prescribed were nontoxic and resulted in benefit. While the case continues to progress at the time of writing this book, just like all treatment plans, the goal is to decrease the amount of dietary supplements at the end of the program and see if the clinical improvement continues. If symptoms regress, then individual agents are added back to the recommendations to maintain the benefits.

Treatment Plan

PURE L-ASPARTIC ACID 500 mg: Take two capsules twice daily.

PURE L-GLUTAMIC ACID 500 mg: Take two capsules twice daily for one month, then two capsules once daily thereafter.

For elevated free radical marker (8-Hydroxy-2-deoxyguanosine):
BUFFERED VITAMIN C 1000 mg: Take two capsules twice daily.

N-ACETYL-CYSTEINE (NAC) 900 mg: Take one capsule daily with food. Take one bottle and then discontinue.

EGCG 250 mg: Take two capsules twice daily.

For CoQ10:
COENZYME Q10 POWDER (orange flavor) 110 gm: Take one bottle and then switch to Coenzyme Q10 100 mg.

For vitamin D:
VITAMIN D3 5000 IU: Take one capsule twice daily with food.

For vitamin E:
VITAMIN E MIXED TOCOPH 400 IU: Take one capsule daily with food.

For magnesium:
REJUVAMAG: Take two capsules each night before bed.

For omega-3 and omega-6 fatty acids:
CARLSON'S COD LIVER OIL: Take two tablespoons daily for two months, then decrease to one tablespoon daily. Keep refrigerated.

EVENING PRIMROSE OIL 500 mg: Take two softgels twice daily or four softgels once daily with a meal.

For multiple vitamin:
SUPREME MULTIVITAMIN (WITHOUT IRON): Take four capsules daily with a meal.

COFACTOR B: Take 1 capsule daily with food.

For ability to produce cellular energy:
MITOFORTE: Take four capsules each morning with breakfast.

For toxic metals:
Initiate calcium-disodium EDTA chelation therapy with a doctor in your area. Referrals will be provided, if necessary.

Chapter Fifteen

Bipolar Disorder

Bipolar disorder, also called manic-depressive illness, is a disorder characterized by dramatic, and sometimes rapid, mood swings. People may go from overly energetic, "highs" and/or irritable, to sad and hopeless, and then back again. They often have normal moods in between. Bipolar disorder can run in families, and people with a first-degree relative (e.g., mother, father, siblings) with this disorder run a seven times greater risk than people in the general population of having bipolar disorder. This disorder usually starts in late adolescence or early adulthood.

Bipolar disorder, or manic-depressive illness, has been recognized since at least the time of Hippocrates, who described such patients as "amic" and "melancholic." In 1899, Emil Kraepelin defined manic-depressive illness and noted that persons with manic-depressive illness lacked deterioration and dementia, which he associated with schizophrenia. Conventional medicine has no explanation of the underlying causes of bipolar disorder.

Dr. Pieczenik

Dr. Pieczenik has had a problem with the diagnosis and treatment of bipolar disease. In his experience starting at St. Elizabeth's Hospital in Washington DC, the original diagnosis of bipolar disorder was schizoaffective disorder, which meant that it was primarily a cognitive disorder with an affective component. At that time it was recognized that there was a disturbance of the neurotransmitter system. Dr. Pieczenik started treating these patients with antipsychotic agents, which ameliorated the problem. Later lithium was introduced as a potential treatment option, and Dr. Pieczenik started prescribing lithium in the hospital setting. Again, the patients improved, but no one on either of these medications was ever cured.

Worse yet, what happened is that Dr. Pieczenik performed autopsies on approximately 10% of the patients who received lithium and found that even with normal serum lithium levels, there were huge deposits of lithium in the heart, kidneys, liver, and nervous system. In effect, Dr. Pieczenik concluded that he was poisoning the patient in an attempt to cure him. Dr. Pieczenik concluded that given the ages at which these patients died that the lithium may have precipitated an earlier death.

Subsequently the diagnosis of schizoaffective disorder changed to manic depressive disorder. Later the diagnosis was again changed to bipolar disorder, which is the common diagnosis now thanks to the current diagnostic criteria, which came from England. In Dr. Pieczenik's belief, the real reason why the cognitive component was removed the diagnosis and it became a strict mood disorder was not because the psychiatric community understood the disease any better or that any new research findings had emerged to redefine this entity, but rather it was simply because the DSM diagnostic criteria were redefined by the pharmaceutical industry so that more drugs could be sold.

These classes of medications that are still being used now are the same ones that were used forty years ago, just in a more refined way. In nearly a half century of so-called medical advances the medical and research community has yet to come out with why any of these medications—antipsychotics, antiepileptics, antidepressants, lithium, or even electroconvulsive therapy (ECT)—works, other than saying, as the drug manufacturers' Web sites state, that the drugs are "believed to work by balancing the chemicals naturally found in the brain."

The bottom line is that no etiology, pathophysiology, or objective biological markers for this condition have been determined. Unfortunately, in the process, many bipolar patients may improve, but the subsequent long-term side effects from these medications are not known. Therefore, it's crucial that another approach to diagnosis and treatment be investigated. Dr. Pieczenik believes that functional medicine and in particular, functional biochemistry, offers this opportunity.

Dr. Neustadt

Just as conventional medicine has no cure for bipolar disorder, naturopathic medicine has no documented cure either. However, there is limited but provocative research documenting that nutritional deficiencies may contribute to bipolar disorder and that nutritional interventions may stabilize mood in these patients, even allowing some of them to discontinue their medications.[255-257] Dr. Neustadt counsels patients to discontinue their medications only after consulting with the physician who prescribed the medication. In the case below, however, this patient came in after suffering from mood cycling for many years without any diagnosis. In addition to Dr. Neustadt's own intake and recommendations, to ensure that the patient was receiving the best possible care, he also referred him to a medical doctor. Dr. Neustadt wanted his colleague to evaluate this patient and perhaps prescribe a medication to stabilize his mood while they were waiting for the patient's MetaCT 400 test results. However, since the medical doctor was familiar with Dr. Neustadt's work, she recommended that the patient first see if Dr. Neustadt could help him before beginning any medications.

The testing and treatment approach in this patient was successful. His mood cycling stopped, and he experienced great benefits in his overall health. The caveat here is that the authors fully realize that the results in this one patient with this approach may not be typical; however, they believe that it generates interesting propositions and possibilities.

Case: Rapid Cycling Bipolar Disorder in a Twenty-five-year-old Man

A twenty-five-year-old man presented to Montana Integrative Medicine for an appointment with Dr. Neustadt. This patient complained of suffering from alternating severe anxiety and depression for the past seven years. Several years earlier his sister was diagnosed with bipolar disorder, and his maternal grandfather suffered from depression and committed suicide. He had tried some natural therapies for his anxiety in the past, including Kava kava, St. John's wort, Yarrow root, and Skullcap. All of these were helpful immediately afterwards, but gave no long-term benefits. Counseling with a therapist did not help. He was prescribed Xanax to help with the anxiety until his test results came back and the underlying biochemical abnormalities could be treated.

Low essential amino acids and elevated ethanolamine, which has been associated with the onset of bipolar disorder and depression

Arginine	58	
Histidine	64	L
Isoleucine	42	L
Leucine	86	L
Lysine	152	
Methionine	32	
Phenylalanine	46	
Threonine	134	
Tryptophan	39	
Valine	147	L
Serine	94	
Taurine	69	
Ethanolamine	10	H

Low minerals (note: magnesium and manganese are required to process and lower the amino acid ethanolamine, above)

Chromium	0.29
Copper	0.63
Magnesium	45
Manganese	0.25

Low omega-3 series polyunsaturated fatty acids

Alpha Linolenic (18:3n3)	9	L
Eicosapentaenoic (20:5n3)	11	L
Docosapentaenoic (22:5n3)	26	
Docosahexaenoic (22:6n3)	31	L

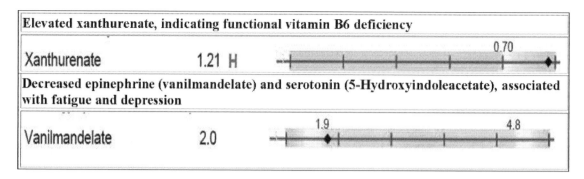

Elevated xanthurenate, indicating functional vitamin B6 deficiency

Xanthurenate	1.21 H

0.70

Decreased epinephrine (vanilmandelate) and serotonin (5-Hydroxyindoleacetate), associated with fatigue and depression

Vanilmandelate	2.0

1.9   4.8

The man was placed on nutraceuticals to correct his underlying biochemical abnormalities. After two weeks on the program he reported feeling "good," and that he had only had one bad day in the past two weeks, which was caused by him not eating and not taking his nutraceuticals. After six weeks on the program, the patient reported that he had not experienced any depression or anxiety for more than a month. He felt his mood was "stable," and his mood was not cycling. All of his symptoms resolved, and after six months, he continued to have no symptoms of bipolar disorder.

* * *

Treatment Plan

This treatment plan is based on your tests and your interview and physical examination with/by Dr. Neustadt. Your tests revealed the following: (1) functional vitamin B6 deficiency, which has been linked to depression, (2) low catecholamines (neurotransmitters), which have been linked to depression and anxiety, (3) low serotonin, which has been linked to depression, anxiety, insomnia, fatigue, constipation, and attention deficit disorder, (4) multiple low minerals, (5) multiple low amino acids, (6) elevated ethanolamine, which has been linked to depression and bipolar disorder, (7) low liver detoxification of sulfur compounds, (8) and low omega-3 essential fatty acids, which has been linked to inflammation and depression.

Dietary supplements:

SUPREME MULTIVITAMIN (WITHOUT IRON): Take four capsules daily with a meal.

PROMINERALS: Take three capsules daily with food. *Take one bottle and then discontinue.*

RESCULPT: Stir or blend two two scoops (23g) of ReSculpt into 8 fl. oz. of water, milk, or juice twice daily.

PERFUSIA-SR: Take two capsules once daily.

N-ACETYL-CYSTEINE (NAC) 1,000 mg: Take one capsule daily with food.

CARLSON'S COD LIVER OIL: Take three tablespoons once daily for two weeks, then two tablespoons daily after that. Note: In rare cases high doses can stimulate a manic episode in people. If this occurs, discontinue the fish oil and call Dr. Neustadt to report this. Also, take this for one month, then decrease to one tablespoon once daily.

FLAX OIL: Continue taking your flax oil you're already taking.

MAG-10: Take one capsule daily with a meal.

MITOFORTE: Take four capsules once daily each morning with a meal.

PURE ORNITHINE-KETOGLUTARATE 500 mg: Take two capsules per day on with water or fruit juice. Do not take with dairy products.

COFACTOR B: Take one capsule daily with food.

Chapter Sixteen

Obesity and Diabetes

Obesity is a dangerous metabolic condition that results in increased risk of diabetes, heart disease, cancer, degenerative joint disease, and premature death. Obesity in the United States has increased at "an epidemic rate" over the last twenty years. The percentage of U.S. adults classified as overweight increased from 56% in 1994 to 65% in 2002, and obesity increased from 23% to 30% during this same time period. Approximately 16% of children and adolescents six to nineteen years old were overweight in 2002.

Obesity is frequently accompanied by diabetes. Diabetes mellitus (diabetes) is a chronic condition that affects over nineteen million Americans. Type 2 diabetes is the most prevalent form, affecting approximately seventeen million individuals. The incidence of type 2 diabetes is growing, with a 49% increase in diagnoses for this condition seen between 1990 and 2000. Type 2 diabetes used to be called adult-onset diabetes and non-insulin dependent diabetes mellitus.

New evidence has made these terms obsolete, as they are no longer adequately descriptive. This is because the disease is no longer primarily limited to adults, with incidence of type 2 diabetes in children skyrocketing. Additionally, if the condition is not controlled, insulin administration is required in the later stages of disease management. Type 2 diabetes is thought to be preceded by a condition known as insulin resistance syndrome or metabolic syndrome. This is a pre-diabetic state that may involve a decrease in the ability of cells to respond to insulin (insulin resistance), a decrease in HDL cholesterol, and an increase in LDL cholesterol, obesity, and high blood pressure.

Case: Obesity and Pre-diabetes in a Fifty-five-year-old Man

This is the case of a fifty-five-year-old man who had been struggling for years spending tens of thousands of dollars on personal trainers and medical testing to improve his health. However, his health continued to deteriorate. He rated his energy at one out of ten (ten being best) and complained of being extremely tired "all the time." He wanted to improve his health but was too fatigued to exercise.

His MetaCT 400 biochemical test panel revealed extremely elevated insulin and fasting blood sugar, inability to produce energy due deficiencies in nutrients required to burn fats and sugars for energy, a raging intestinal fungal infection (candidiasis), and allergies to eighteen different common foods such as garlic, eggs, dairy, and almonds. Eating foods to which people are allergic causes a chronic inflammation in the gut that can decrease the ability to digest and absorb nutrients, predispose someone to intestinal infections, cause malnutrition, and set someone up for long-term, degenerative diseases such as diabetes and obesity.

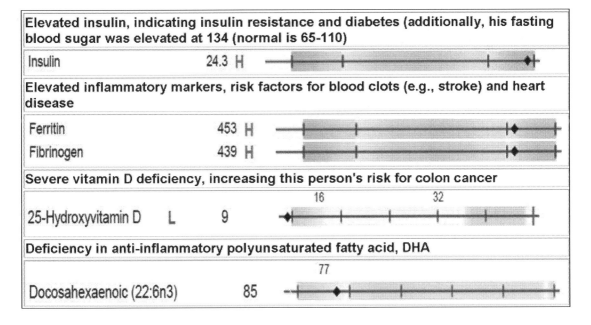

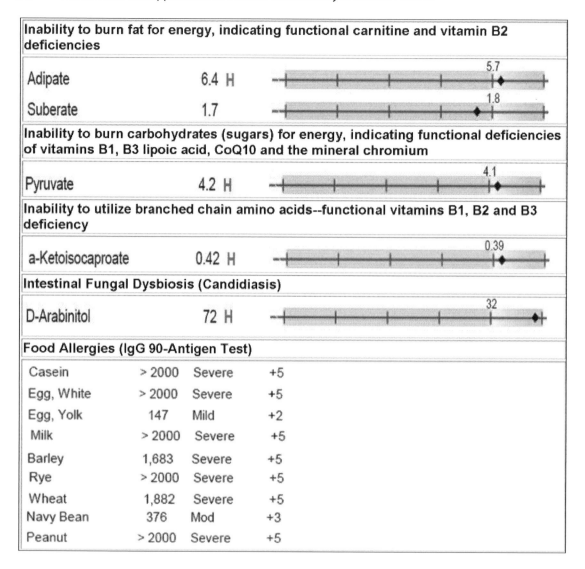

Inability to burn fat for energy, indicating functional carnitine and vitamin B2 deficiencies		
Adipate	6.4 H	5.7
Suberate	1.7	1.8
Inability to burn carbohydrates (sugars) for energy, indicating functional deficiencies of vitamins B1, B3 lipoic acid, CoQ10 and the mineral chromium		
Pyruvate	4.2 H	4.1
Inability to utilize branched chain amino acids--functional vitamins B1, B2 and B3 deficiency		
a-Ketoisocaproate	0.42 H	0.39
Intestinal Fungal Dysbiosis (Candidiasis)		
D-Arabinitol	72 H	32
Food Allergies (IgG 90-Antigen Test)		
Casein	> 2000	Severe	+5
Egg, White	> 2000	Severe	+5
Egg, Yolk	147	Mild	+2
Milk	> 2000	Severe	+5
Barley	1,683	Severe	+5
Rye	> 2000	Severe	+5
Wheat	1,882	Severe	+5
Navy Bean	376	Mod	+3
Peanut	> 2000	Severe	+5

This gentleman was placed on an aggressive plan of dietary modification, exercise, and dietary supplements to help correct his biochemical abnormalities, decrease his weight, and restore his health. He worked with a nutritionist and exercised regularly. After three months, a retest of his fasting insulin showed that it had decreased by 50% (see below), and he had also decreased his waistline by two pant sizes.

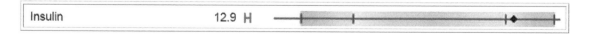

Insulin	12.9 H	

Over time, this person will likely be able to reintroduce some of the foods to which he was allergic, but only after following a gut restoration program intended to rid the intestines of the fungal overgrowth, decrease the inflammation, and heal and cells lining the intestinal tract. However, the take-home message here is that through a simple, customized approach to health care based on testing the underlying biochemical abnormalities creating the disease, it's quite easy to improve one's health. What people need first, however, are the data to create the plan, which are provided through testing.

* * *

Treatment Plan

Diet:
AVOID all *casein (a protein in dairy and dairy products), dairy and dairy products, eggs, and egg-containing products, barley, rye, wheat, peanut, navy beans, malt, almonds, cashews, pistachios, sunflower (an sunflower oil), mustard greens, and garlic* for eight weeks, then reintroduce them into your diet.

For intestinal bacterial and fungal overgrowth:
NYSTATIN TABLETS, 500,000 units twice daily for three months.

BERBERINE FORTE: Take one capsule twice daily with food. Take four bottles of this and then discontinue.

ENTEROPRO: Take one capsule daily with food.

For elevated cardiovascular risk factors:
FENUCHROME: Take three capsules once daily with food.

PROTECT DM: Take one capsule daily.

NATTOPINE: Take two capsules daily.

NIASAFE: Take two capsules twice daily.

For gut healing:
GLUTAMINE RX: Mix one teaspoon twice daily in water and drink.

For elevated ADMA and blood pressure:

PERFUSIA SR: Take three capsules twice daily.

For vitamin and mineral insufficiencies:

Intravenous nutritional drips and intramuscular vitamin D shots twice weekly for two weeks, then weekly thereafter for another six weeks.

SUPREME MULTIVITAMIN (WITHOUT IRON): Take four capsules daily with a meal.

MITOFORTE: Take two capsules each morning with breakfast.

Chapter Seventeen

Neustadt-Pieczenik Athlete's Depletion Syndrome (ADS)

The Neustadt-Pieczenik Athlete's Depletion Syndrome (ADS) is characteristic of many people who exert themselves physically and particularly seen in competitive athletes, whom Dr. Neustadt has treated. The history of enhancing performance in athletes with the use of anabolic steroids ("doping") is well known. But the use of these anabolic steroids masks much more serious problems and likely exacerbates by allowing athletes to continue to compete beyond their biochemical and physiological capacity. In short, more athletes who train extensively are often training into what the authors call Athlete's Depletion Syndrome, where the entire spectrum of amino acids, fatty acids, vitamins, and minerals are seriously depleted, leading to blood sugar dysregulation, lipids dysregulation, and decreased ability to utilize nutrients for cellular energy. This leads to muscle wasting, depression, insomnia, and complete physical and mental exhaustion.

By masking these problems, it turns into a vicious cycle. The athlete pushes him or herself harder and harder to compensate for decreased performance and capability. What happens in athletic training for most of these athletes is that they overstress the body and the mind. At the time of competition, the body and mind must react with a spontaneous agility that's not normal. In this case, because of the training and lack of understanding of the underlying functional biochemistry of the training, when you look at their analytes, their profiles are very consistent. Namely, they experience depletions of amino acids, vitamins, minerals, and fats, with all the concomitant symptoms of insomnia, irritability, and blood sugar dysregulation. This pattern actually closely resembles Age-Related Degeneration (ARD), in which the elderly have panoply of deficiencies and symptoms, but the cause is different.

This cycle in athletic performance is improved by letting them rest and through attempts to optimize their diets. However, in a subset of athletes whose performance is declining and who are exhibiting the characteristic symptoms of ADS, these approaches are inadequate and compound the problem even further. They are in a downward spiral so severely that eventually their body is literally destroying itself, such as catabolizing muscle to maintain circulating amino acid pools for use in hormones and other systems.

These athletes are so primed for athletic performance and competing to win that if they are off by even a millisecond, they can go into a depression. These depressions can be quite severe and are compounded by the physiological degeneration. While giving them antidepressants or performance-enhancing drugs may improve their mood and even their performance, it masks an insidious and worsening underlying fundamental problem of catabolism.

Case: ADS in a Seventeen-year-old Female High School Athlete

The mother of a seventeen-year-old girl made an appointment for her daughter with Dr. Neustadt in a desperate attempt to stop her daughter's deteriorating condition. The girl was on the local high school track team. She had many primary complaints. She had been suffering with depression, for which she took 10 mg of Prozac daily. Her energy was five out of ten, with ten being best, for the past three years. She suffered from sleep phase delay and sleep phase advance and would wake up one to five times each night. This disordered sleep pattern had been going on for "years."

A review of symptoms revealed that the girl was suffering from orthostatic hypotension three time daily, bilateral knee and ankle pain for the past five years, which had progressed to the point that she couldn't participate in the sports she loved, such as track and skiing. For years she had been experiencing bilateral frontal headaches three times each that were not progressing and did not cause any visual disturbances. She had post-nasal drip "all the time" for years and suffered from gas and bloating three times each week. She also mentioned that she had brain fog, with difficulty processing information. She had heavy and long menstrual bleeding, for which she was seeing her family physician. She had food cravings for sugar and complained also of binge eating, lack of endurance, apathy, leg cramps, dark circles under her eyes, and water retention.

Her MetaCT 400 test results revealed:

Moderate and severe food allergies			
Egg, White	576	Mod	+4
Egg, Yolk	1,200	Severe	+5
Navy Bean	236	Mod	+3
Pinto Bean	458	Mod	+3
Ginger	342	Mod	+3

Amino acid deficiencies leading to muscle catabolism, blood sugar dysregulation, depression and, in the case of low proline, increased osteoporosis risk, a symptom of the Athlete's Triad. This also indicates decreased exercise tolerance and stamina.

Amino Acid	Value	
Isoleucine	57	
Arginine	49	L
Histidine	77	
Phenylalanine	43	L
Threonine	103	
Leucine	108	
Tryptophan	37	
Lysine	137	L
Methionine	24	L
Valine	212	
Glycine	224	L
Serine	91	
Tyrosine	49	L
Taurine	43	L
Asparagine	54	
Aspartic Acid	5.7	L
Citrulline	28	
Glutamic Acid	36	L
Glutamine	626	
Ornithine	46	L
a-Aminoadipic Acid	2.6	
Proline	116	L
Alanine	250	

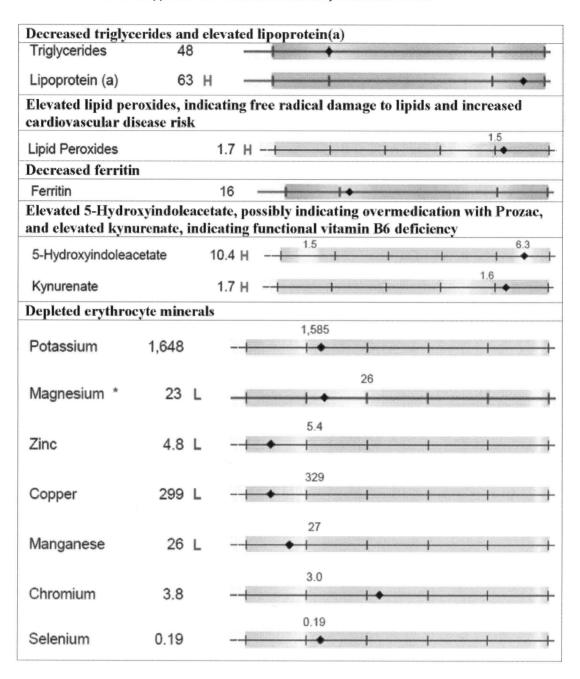

Decreased triglycerides and elevated lipoprotein(a)		
Triglycerides	48	
Lipoprotein (a)	63 H	

Elevated lipid peroxides, indicating free radical damage to lipids and increased cardiovascular disease risk

Lipid Peroxides	1.7 H	1.5

Decreased ferritin

Ferritin	16	

Elevated 5-Hydroxyindoleacetate, possibly indicating overmedication with Prozac, and elevated kynurenate, indicating functional vitamin B6 deficiency

5-Hydroxyindoleacetate	10.4 H	1.5 6.3
Kynurenate	1.7 H	1.6

Depleted erythrocyte minerals

Potassium	1,648	1,585
Magnesium *	23 L	26
Zinc	4.8 L	5.4
Copper	299 L	329
Manganese	26 L	27
Chromium	3.8	3.0
Selenium	0.19	0.19

Depleted omega-3, omega-6 and saturated fatty acids, putting her at risk for amenorrhea, one symptom of the Athlete's Triad

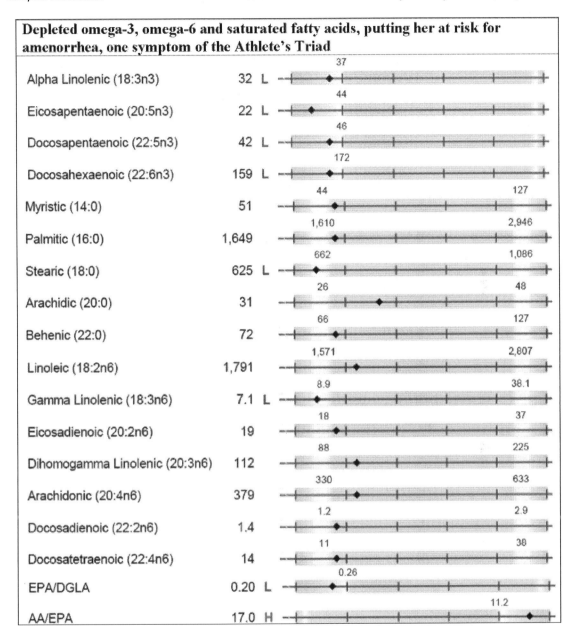

Alpha Linolenic (18:3n3)	32 L	37
Eicosapentaenoic (20:5n3)	22 L	44
Docosapentaenoic (22:5n3)	42 L	46
Docosahexaenoic (22:6n3)	159 L	172
Myristic (14:0)	51	44 — 127
Palmitic (16:0)	1,649	1,610 — 2,946
Stearic (18:0)	625 L	662 — 1,086
Arachidic (20:0)	31	26 — 48
Behenic (22:0)	72	66 — 127
Linoleic (18:2n6)	1,791	1,571 — 2,807
Gamma Linolenic (18:3n6)	7.1 L	8.9 — 38.1
Eicosadienoic (20:2n6)	19	18 — 37
Dihomogamma Linolenic (20:3n6)	112	88 — 225
Arachidonic (20:4n6)	379	330 — 633
Docosadienoic (22:2n6)	1.4	1.2 — 2.9
Docosatetraenoic (22:4n6)	14	11 — 38
EPA/DGLA	0.20 L	0.26
AA/EPA	17.0 H	11.2

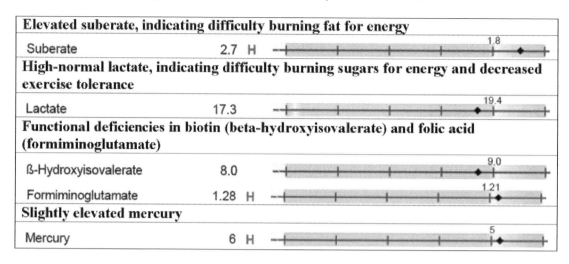

Elevated suberate, indicating difficulty burning fat for energy		
Suberate	2.7 H	1.8
High-normal lactate, indicating difficulty burning sugars for energy and decreased exercise tolerance		
Lactate	17.3	19.4
Functional deficiencies in biotin (beta-hydroxyisovalerate) and folic acid (formiminoglutamate)		
ß-Hydroxyisovalerate	8.0	9.0
Formiminoglutamate	1.28 H	1.21
Slightly elevated mercury		
Mercury	6 H	5

* * *

Treatment Plan

Diet:

AVOID all *eggs and all egg-containing products, ginger, pinto beans, and navy beans* for eight weeks, and then reintroduce them into your diet.

For amino acids:

CUSTOMIZED AMINO ACID BLEND: Take as directed on the bottle.

GLYCINE POWDER: Mix ½ teaspoon daily with water with or between meals. Take one bottle of this and then discontinue.

GLUTAMINE RX: Mix one teaspoon twice daily in water and drink.

For elevated lipoprotein(a) and lipid peroxides:

BUFFERED VITAMIN C 1,000 mg: Take three capsules daily, all in divided doses.

CURCUMIN PRO 450 mg: Take one tablet twice daily.

PROTECT DM: Take one capsule daily.

For iron deficiency (low ferritin; your goal for ferritin is 90–110):

FERROSOLVE: Take one capsule daily with or without food.

For low minerals:

PROMINERALS: Take three capsules daily with food. Take two bottles and then discontinue.

REJUVAMAG: Take one capsule each night before bed.

SUPREME FEM MULTIVITAMIN (WITH IRON): Take four capsules daily with a meal.

For fatty acids:

CARLSON'S COD LIVER OIL: Take one tablespoon (equivalent of three teaspoons) twice daily for one month, then one tablespoon daily thereafter. Keep refrigerated.

For ability to burn fats for energy:

MITOFORTE: Take four capsules each morning with breakfast.

For biotin:

BIOTIN 5000 MCG: Take one capsule daily.

For folic acid:

FA-8 FOLIC ACID 800 mcg: Take one capsule daily.

For mercury toxicity:

Consider toxic metals chelation therapy. Discuss this with Dr. Neustadt.

For knee pain:

PROLOTHERAPY injections to both knees, spaced four to six weeks apart. A series of four to six injections is recommended, and then we will reevaluate.

* * *

In addition to the treatment plan, Dr. Neustadt requested this girl not join the track team this year and abstain from any exercise for three months, except for walking or light bike riding. This recommendation was made in order to decrease the stress on her body and give it time to recover. Over the course of the three-month treatment plan, this girl's depression lifted, and she was weaned off her Prozac. The dark circles under her eyes disappeared, her energy increased to seven to eight out of ten with ten being best, her headaches decreased by 30%, she no longer had any orthostatic hypotension, the post-nasal drip completely resolved, as did the gas and bloating. Her brain fog improved by 90%, her sugar cravings went away, as did her binge eating, apathy, and leg cramps.

One aspect of the treatment plan that she struggled with was improving her sleep. Most of the clinical signs improved rapidly; however, her energy and brain fog did not improve until her sleep was better regulated. In this case merely practicing "sleep hygiene" and consuming five grams of protein at bedtime did not work. Not until her mother purchased Night Rest, a sleep dietary supplement by Source Naturals, did her sleep improve, and with it the final, recalcitrant symptoms. At the time of writing this book the patient had still not undergone prolotherapy treatments, and her joint pains had not improved.

Chapter Eighteen

Pulmonary Infections

Medicine approaches pulmonary diseases in a very linear fashion. Basically, pulmonology evaluates lung capacity through spirometry testing. Based on the test results, most pulmonary conditions are divided into two categories: (1) restrictive diseases, and (2) obstructive disorders. The categories of pulmonary diseases include: airway disorders (e.g., asthma), interstitial lung disease, alveolar space disease, pulmonary vasculature diseases, pleural diseases, disorders of ventilator control, environmental diseases, infectious lung disease, and malignant neoplastic lung disease.

The diagnostic capabilities in pulmonary medicine far outweigh the capacity to treat the pulmonary diseases. If it's a reactive airway disorder, such as asthma, doctors prescribe a bronchodilator and a steroid. This has not changed in forty to fifty years. If it's an infection, the organism may be cultured via sputum, lung aspiration, or lung biopsy, and is treated with an appropriate antimicrobial medication.

This sounds pretty straightforward: identify the cause of a symptom and treat it. However, this approach, while helpful and even life-saving in some cases, can be severely lacking in other cases. Often people can become addicted to an inhalator, even when it ceases to be a helpful medication. People can also become resistant to steroids, which requires ever higher doses and increases their risk of osteoporosis and other side effects. And in chronic pulmonary infections, repeated antimicrobial medications do not actually kill the organisms and restore health. So the notion that people can breathe more easily as advertised by the pharmaceutical industry on television is a misleading one.

Dr. Neustadt has documented successes with the functional biochemistry approach in chronic pulmonary infections and asthma, as demonstrated by several cases.

Case: Seven-year Intractable Pulmonary Infections

This case is an interesting one because it illustrates the many important features of physician-patient and physician-physician relationships, as well as the complexity of the problem itself. It also demonstrates the power of a targeted approach to complex conditions based on functional biochemical testing instead of a shotgun approach based on symptoms.

Dr. Pieczenik

It also illustrates that a naturopathic physician can take a very complex medical problem that has been evaluated and treated for over seven years without success, and first of all, not be intimidated by the complexity of the problem. Second, this type of problem would always be handled by the pulmonary and/or infectious disease departments of a major medical institution. Very rarely would it ever be handed over to an internist or a family practitioner. And it would never be referred to a naturopathic doctor. But in this particular case the approach that Dr. Neustadt took was one of trying to kill the infection while simultaneously improving the immune system. From the medical perspective, this approach would never have been taken.

The infectious disease that was diagnosed would have been compounded by iatrogenic complications. This in turn would compound the problem of infectious diseases in general without ever resolving the underlying problem of what was wrong with her total body physiology and biochemistry that would predispose her to recurrent infections. At no point would any medical doctor consider the notion of nutrition, diet, and lifestyle, other than to suggest that the patient not smoke or live in a humid environment. Therefore, the conventional medical approach would be to target the specific organism that was cultured out at any particular time. In short, allopathic medicine approached this complicated problem very simplistically, despite the fact that medicine sees itself as very sophisticated, strategic, and frequently the arbiter of a complex set of knowledge unavailable to the lay person.

Microbial culture and sensitivity led to antibiotic treatments. Inflammation and bronchoconstriction leads to bronchodilators and steroids. What was constricted were not only the bronchi, but the conventional medical mindset, be it internal medicine, infectious diseases or pulmonology.

Dr. Neustadt

Most of the patients who end up in Dr. Neustadt's office have been suffering for years with chronic, debilitating conditions that are only getting worse. They have been through the conventional medical system without benefit. These patients are seeking an evidence-based, scientifically rigorous alternative approach. Drs. Piezenik and Neustadt often call this phenomenon the "medicine of desperation" or the "medicine of last resort."

From a naturopathic perspective, many infectious diseases are opportunistic diseases. Many people are exposed to the same organism, but not everyone gets sick. Working with infectious diseases then requires a three-pronged approach: (1) kill the organism with antimicrobials; (2) remove any influences that decrease immune function, such as food allergies, stress and subclinical nutritional deficiencies; and (3) boost immune function through dietary and lifestyle changes and dietary supplements. In the two pulmonary infections cases illustrated here, this approach worked better than the conventional medical approach. This is not to say that the conventional approach should be abandoned, or cannot improve patients' health by narrowly evaluating and treating the infections; however, in these cases the conventional approach was incomplete and unfortunately, downright ineffectual.

HISTORY OF PRESENT ILLNESS: The patient comes in today complaining of multiple lung infections with difficulty breathing and fatigue. Onset was 1999 when she was diagnosed with "hot tub syndrome." This syndrome results from a weakened immune system, which she experienced with bronchitis prior to going on vacation and spending hours and hours in a hot tub. At that time she contracted mycobacterium avium complex (MAC) infection. She has has never smoked.

She has been hospitalized five times since 1999, with recurrent Stevens-Johnson Syndrome. She experienced these Stevens-Johnson Syndrome episodes while not taking any medication. She has a history of taking chlorythromycin and clofazamine for two years. She was recently diagnosed by a pulmonologist with a *Paecilomyces* infection. In May 2006 she was diagnosed with a *Citrobacter* infection. She currently has sinusitis. She has also been diagnosed with Lady

Windemere Syndrome, manifesting as a decreased cough reflex. She also reports having silent aspiration and recurrent bronchitis.

For these complaints she has tried several different alternative medicines in the past. For instance, acupuncture increased her energy but had no change on the cough. She has tried homeopathy. She has tried various herbs including one "lung formula." She hangs upside down "to move stuff around." She complains of phlegm pooling in her lungs and hanging upside down helps to relieve the pressure of that and expel the phlegm. She has also tried huff coughing.

SOCIAL AND FAMILY HISTORY: The patient is a mother of three children, ages twelve, ten, and eight.

PAST MEDICAL HISTORY: She has a significant medical history for multiple pulmonary infections and other pathologies: MAC diagnosed in 1999. Bronchiectasis diagnosed in 1999. Pneumonia in 2005. She was hospitalized five times for Stevens-Johnson Syndrome in 1999 while not taking any medications. She had chest x-rays done which showed "white spots" on her lungs. In 2006 she was diagnosed with a *Paecilomyces* infection. Her CT scans have not found any indication of fungi per her report.

CURRENT MEDICATIONS: Clofazamine 50mg twice daily for the past two years. Chlorythromycin 250mg three times daily for the past two years. Advair for the past four years. Levaquin 500mg daily for the past two weeks. Clindamycin 400mg three times daily for the past two weeks. Mytussin AC syrup one to two teaspoons as needed for the past three days. Levaquin, clindamycin, and Mytussin AC syrup are all short-term treatments, according to the patient, which she will discontinue shortly. Note: Patient had been prescribed steroids in the past, which she reported triggered a "psychosis reaction."

DIETARY SUPPLEMENTS: The patient is taking a multiple vitamin and a probiotic.

SLEEP: She sleeps six to eight hours a day. No sleep phase delay or sleep phase advance. She wakes refreshed.

ENERGY: two out of ten, ten being best. Her energy range is from zero to four out of ten. The energy being two out of ten has been going on for two months, at which time her coughing started to get worse again.

STRESS: two out of ten, ten being the worst.

DIET RECALL: Breakfast—she was not hungry today. She had one grain of whole grain toast, water, and tea; Lunch—half of an avocado and a piece of cheese; Dinner—ratatouille, wine, and ice cream; Cravings—none; Snacks—"not much."

REVIEW OF SYSTEMS: No weight changes. Patient reports frequent fevers. She is experiencing brain fog secondary to sinus congestion, per her report. She is experiencing dysphagia. She had a barium swallow done which showed "swallowing not very good." She is experiencing "a sensation like her chest is full of concrete." According to the patient, this is secondary to the accumulation of phlegm and her decreased ability to get full breaths of air. Her dyspnea would trigger panic attacks. She is not having any sharp chest pains. She is experiencing gas and bloating. No belching. No abdominal pains. No discomfort. No feeling of quick fullness after eating. She is having a bowel movement on most days. She has no undigested food in her stool. Her urine is okay—no dysuria, no urgency, no post-void dribbling. She is experiencing numbness in her toes and fingers, which comes and goes. She is also experiencing trembling in her hands which has been going on for the past two months. She reports that when she gets sick, she always gets trembling. She is also suffering from frequent muscle cramps.

PHYSICAL EXAMINATION: The patient was very friendly and animated during today's conversation. She is eager to get a second opinion on what she might be able to try to boost her immune system. She was alert and oriented times three and in no acute distress. General—Wt: 125lbs. Ht: 5'4" Temp: 98.4°F BP: 112/76 Pulse: 76 bpm and full. ENT—Trachea midline. No submandibular, submental or cervical chain lymphadenopathy. Tympanic membranes were visible bilaterally and displayed no erythema. She has no erythema in her posterior pharynx. Her maxillary sinuses were tender to palpation bilaterally. Lungs—Inspiratory and expiratory wheezes heard in all lung fields.

Her MetaCT 400 test results showed:

Low CoQ10		
Coenzyme Q10	0.44 L	
Low minerals		
Copper	0.54	
Magnesium	45	
Vanadium	0.11	
Zinc	6.4	
Vitamin D insufficiency		
25-hydroxyvitamin D	28	
Low omega-3 fatty acids		
Alpha Linolenic (18:3n3)	19	
Eicosapentaenoic (20:5n3)	24	
Docosapentaenoic (22:5n3)	25	
Docosahexaenoic (22:6n3)	83	
Decreased ability to burn sugars for cellular energy		
Pyruvate	3.6	
Lactate	16.2	
ß-Hydroxybutyrate	4.5 H	
Multiple blockages in Kreb's Cycle intermediates required for cellular energy production		
Citrate	1,220 H	
Succinate	30.3 H	
Fumarate	4.54 H	
Malate	3.7 H	
Hydroxymethylglutarate	10.9 H	

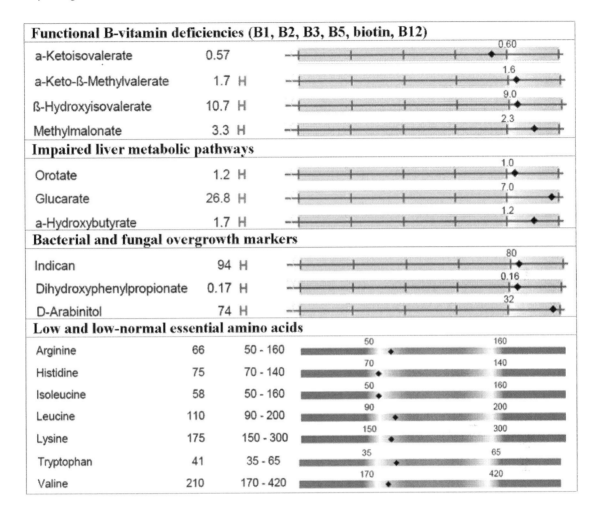

Functional B-vitamin deficiencies (B1, B2, B3, B5, biotin, B12)		
a-Ketoisovalerate	0.57	0.60
a-Keto-ß-Methylvalerate	1.7 H	1.6
ß-Hydroxyisovalerate	10.7 H	9.0
Methylmalonate	3.3 H	2.3
Impaired liver metabolic pathways		
Orotate	1.2 H	1.0
Glucarate	26.8 H	7.0
a-Hydroxybutyrate	1.7 H	1.2
Bacterial and fungal overgrowth markers		
Indican	94 H	80
Dihydroxyphenylpropionate	0.17 H	0.16
D-Arabinitol	74 H	32

Low and low-normal essential amino acids			
Arginine	66	50 - 160	50 / 160
Histidine	75	70 - 140	70 / 140
Isoleucine	58	50 - 160	50 / 160
Leucine	110	90 - 200	90 / 200
Lysine	175	150 - 300	150 / 300
Tryptophan	41	35 - 65	35 / 65
Valine	210	170 - 420	170 / 420

* * *

Treatment Plan

This treatment plan is based on your NBI Testing and Consulting test results, your medical history, and your health goals as discussed with Dr. Neustadt. Your labs revealed: (1) amino acid deficiencies; (2) elevated cardiovascular disease risk factors; (3) antioxidant vitamin deficiency (specifically, CoQ10); (4) mineral deficiencies; (5) elevated free radical damage to DNA (elevated 8-Hydroxy-2-deoxyguanosine); (6) low vitamin D2; (7) low omega-3 series polyunsaturated fatty acids; (8) multiple functional nutritional deficiencies, including

B-vitamins, carnitine, chromium, and lipoic acid; (9) intestinal bacterial and fungal infections; (10) elevated fasting blood sugar.

For intestinal fungal overgrowth:
NYSTATIN TABLETS, 500,000 units twice daily for three months.

For intestinal bacterial overgrowth:
BERBERINE FORTE: Take one capsule twice daily with food.

ENTEROPRO: Take one capsule daily with food.

For vitamin and mineral deficiencies:
SUPREME FEM MULTIVITAMIN (WITH IRON): Take four capsules daily with a meal.

PROMINERALS: Take three capsules daily with food. Take one bottle and then discontinue.

SUPER D3: Take two capsules daily with food.

MITOFORTE: Take four capsules each morning.

COFACTOR B: Take one capsule daily with food.

MAG-10: Take one capsule daily with a meal.

REJUVAMAG: Take two capsules each night before bed.

VITAMIN C POWDER: Mix one scoop twice daily in water, and drink with a meal.

For low amino acids:
Note: All powders can be combined and taken at the same time if desired.

RESCULPT: Stir or blend two scoops (23g) of ReSculpt into 8 fl. oz. of water, milk, or juice once daily.

TAURINE POWDER: Take 1/2 teaspoon daily on an empty stomach (thirty minutes before eating or 1.5 hours after eating).

Specific formula for blood sugar control:
FENUCHROME: Take three capsules once daily with food.

* * *

Two weeks after beginning the program, the patient returned for her first follow up. She was complying with the program and reported that in the intervening two weeks all of her children had the flu. She contracted a "head cold," but the infection did not turn into a respiratory infection. Before she began the treatment plan, she stated that 99.9% of the time the infections would go to her lungs. She went skiing and found that it was like a "normal ski day." Before starting the program, she could only do four runs before she had to quit with exhaustion and shortness of breath. She had not experienced any panic attacks due to dyspnea.

At her six-week follow-up appointment, she reported that she had not had any pulmonary infections since beginning the program. She had an elective surgery ordered by the pulmonologist to biopsy her lung, which did not reveal any conclusive or helpful data. She reported that her "vitality" had increased and that the treatment plan is "giving me the ability to fight back." Her energy had increased to six out of ten, with ten being best (before the treatment plan her energy was two out of ten).

At her three-month follow-up appointment on June 4, 2007, she had an upper respiratory infection, but was able to fight it off without antibiotics. Her energy was seven out of ten, with ten being best. And she reported feeling excellent.

Dr. Neustadt placed her on a maintenance program with minimal dietary supplement support. The patient was lost to follow-up until December 7, 2007, when she came to the clinic reporting a recent diagnosis of pneumonia.

She had previously decided to discontinue all Dr. Neustadt's recommendations because she had been feeling so well, but did not discuss this with Dr. Neustadt first. This illustrates a problem with compliance with patients, who believe that they can manage themselves. In some cases they in fact can manage themselves once the analysis, diagnosis, and treatments are completed. However, Dr. Neustadt has found that closer long-term monitoring is necessary with these chronic infectious diseases.

On December 7, 2007, the patient reported that she had had two rounds of antibiotics since July, 2007, which was "good." She presented with a wet cough and was completing one seven-day round of Levaquin. Her pulmonologist recommended that she return to see Dr. Neustadt because of the extreme benefit she had previously experienced while working with Dr. Neustadt, and because the only treatments the pulmonologist could offer were repeated courses of antibiotics. Dr. Neustadt reviewed her old biochemical test results and placed her on a maintenance program, which was:

Treatment Plan

Intravenous:

I recommend four treatments with medium dose vitamin C (25 g) and supportive nutrients (b-vitamins, minerals). Duration of intravenous drip is approximately 2.513 hours per treatment.

For upper respiratory infection:

URI FORMULA: Take one capsule with a small amount of water three to four times daily between meals.

BERBERINE FORTE: Take one capsule twice daily with food.

ENTEROPRO: Take one capsule daily with food.

For amino acids:

Go to a local health food store and purchase a protein powder you can tolerate that provides about 20 grams of protein per serving. Take once daily.

For vitamin and mineral deficiencies:

SUPREME FEM MULTIVITAMIN (WITH IRON): Take four capsules daily with a meal.

MITOFORTE: Take four capsules each morning with breakfast.

COFACTOR B: Take one capsule daily with food.

MAG-10: Take one capsule daily with a meal.

COENZYME Q10 POWDER 250 mg: Take two scoops dissolved in eight ounces of water daily.

BUFFERED VITAMIN C 1,000 mg: Take four to eight capsules daily, all in divided doses. If diarrhea develops, decrease dose.

N-ACETYL-CYSTEINE (NAC) 1,000 mg: Take one capsule twice daily with food.

GLYCINE POWDER: Mix ½ teaspoon daily at bedtime.

* * *

The patient began the treatment plan and did not return for a follow-up appointment. On September 3, 2008, Dr. Neustadt called her to check on her. The patient reported that prior to starting to work with Dr. Neustadt she was continuously on antibiotics since her initial diagnosis in 1999. As soon as she would stop an antibiotic, she would end up with another infection and get hospitalized. She continued to take her Advair as needed, but all follow-up sputum cultures were negative, without any infections being detected.

The patient began her treatment plan on February 16, 2007. Since beginning the treatment plan, which was subsequently scaled back after three months to a limited maintenance plan, the patient had only had to take two short courses of antibiotics for minor respiratory infections. She had been getting her sputum cultured about 1.5 times every month while being treated by her pulmonologist. Since working with Dr. Neustadt, her sputum cultures had repeatedly come back negative.

Case: Allergic Bronchopulmonary Aspergillosis (ABPA)

A fifty-year-old woman was evaluated by Dr. Neustadt in January 2008. She had been diagnosed with allergic bronchopulmonary aspergillosis (ABPA) in 2004. ABPA is considered a fungal cause of extrinsic eosinophilic syndrome. This syndrome is an immunologic response to *Aspergillus* antigens in the airways. Both IgE-mediated and immune complex-mediated hypersensitivity responses are active. Chemokines recruit CD4+ T helper 2 antigen-specific cells to the lung. The inflammatory responses lead to airway reactivity, mucus hypersecretion, epithelial damage, bronchiectasis, eosinophilic pneumonia, and parenchymal injury and fibrosis. *Aspergillus* proteases likely also contribute to airway damage. Other fungi have also been found to cause a similar disorder, prompting some to suggest renaming this disorder allergic bronchopulmonary mycosis.

She had been placed on multiple rounds of antifungal and antibiotic medications, without any overall benefit. On her Montana Integrative Medicine clinic intake form she wrote that a new problem area was spotted on a recent X-ray on her right lung and that there was a "lack of medical choices in treating ABPA." She wanted to know if there was anything else that could kill the fungus to if Dr. Neustadt could help her resolve her "health challenges."

Dr. Neustadt ordered a MetaCT 150 test, which showed:

Functional deficiencies in the Kreb's Cycle, leading to decreased ability to produce cellular energy			
a-Ketoglutarate	31.0 H		27.8
Succinate	10.5		12.3
Malate	2.6 H		2.3
Functional Vitamin B12 deficiency			
Methylmalonate	2.6 H		2.3
IgG Food Allergies			
Casein	1,764	Severe	+5
Egg, White	963	Severe	+5
Egg, Yolk	684	Mod	+4
Milk	1,048	Severe	+5
Trout	352	Mod	+3
Mustard	597	Mod	+4

* * *

Prior to receiving the test results, Dr. Neustadt prescribed nebulized Fluconazole 1% (10 mg/mL) solution from a compounding pharmacy and instructed her to inhale two mL via a nebulizer twice daily for two months, and to take one bottle of URI Formula, a dietary supplement containing antimicrobial herbs.

Once the MetaCT 150 test results came back, Dr. Neustadt prescribed the following treatment plan in addition to the nebulized Fluconazole. Note: On her subsequent treatment plan, as many liquid and powder forms of nutrients were prescribed as possible, since the patient had a difficult time taking pills.

Treatment Plan

Diet:

AVOID all *egg, egg products, dairy, dairy products, casein (a protein found in high concentrations in dairy and used as a food additive), trout and mustard* for eight weeks, then reintroduce them into your diet.

For intestinal dysbiosis (overgrowth of bacteria and yeast):

BERBERINE FORTE: Take one capsule twice daily with food.

ENTEROPRO: Take one capsule daily with food. Keep refrigerated.

For amino acids (you may mix the powders and take them at the same time):

GLUTAMINE RX: Mix one teaspoon twice daily in water and drink.

BCAA POWDER: Take one scoop per day in a liquid of your choosing.

To burn fat and sugars for cellular energy and to boost your immune system:

EXTREME SPORTS DRINK: Take 1.5 scoops daily (all at once or in divided doses) in water or a beverage of your choice.

ALPHA LIPOIC ACID: Take two capsules daily.

CHEWQ 100 mg: Chew one chewtab with or after a meal.

For vitamin B12 deficiency:

B-12 SUBLINGUAL: Dissolve one lozenge under the tongue daily.

For elevated free radical damage:

CURCUMIN PRO: Take one tablet twice daily.

To increase glutathione:

N-ACETYL-CYSTEINE (NAC) 1,000 mg: Take one capsule daily with food.

For vitamins and minerals:

SUPREME FEM MULTIVITAMIN (WITH IRON): Take four capsules daily with a meal.

VITAMIN D3—continue taking three drops of the liquid vitamin D3, totaling 6,000 IU daily.

For calcium:
CALCIUM (MCHA), 300 mg: Take two capsules daily.

* * *

At her appointment one month later, she reported "feeling well." Her energy was seven out of ten, with ten being best. At her first appointment she reported that her energy was just three out of ten, with ten being best. The patient would use her peak flow meter daily to monitor her air flow. The morning of her appointment with Dr. Neustadt, she reported that her peak flow was 450, whereas it usually was 425. Her sleep had improved. She was sleeping longer without waking up. When she did wake up during the night she could fall back to sleep quicker than before. She was waking up more refreshed each morning. The frequency of coughing up sputum had decreased from daily to just five to six times during the previous month. Her brain fog had improved as well. At that appointment she appeared more animated and conversational. Her physical examination revealed that all lung fields were clear to auscultation. Follow up lung X-rays revealed no consolidation or any pathology.

After three months on the treatment plan, the patient reported that she experienced occasional slight coughing, but without ever coughing up any sputum. She had been able to decrease her Azmacort medication to every other day. Her peak flow was averaging 400, and she was feeling "very good" and had no complaints. Her periorbital edema and allergic shiners had both resolved. She was instructed to follow up as needed.

The patient requested Dr. Neustadt send a chart summary to her pulmonologist, which he did, and which is below.

Chart Summary

Date: May 21, 2008

To: Her Pulmonologist
Fax: xxx-xxx-xxxx

Patient: xx
DOB: x/xx/1957

The patient requested I draft a chart summary for her and send it to her pulmonologist. She originally came to see me on 1/10/2008 for an evaluation of allergic bronchopulmonary aspergillosis (ABPA), which was diagnosed in 2004. She appears to have contracted a pulmonary infection in 2003 while living in Belgium, where she stayed in a "damp church." I confirmed the diagnosis by reviewing the pulmonologist's chart notes and radiology reports brought in by the patient.

The patient also had a history of asthma (diagnosed in 1957), allergies (diagnosed 1957), eczema (diagnosed 1957), *Candida albicans* infection (diagnosed 1990), hypothyroidism (diagnosed 2004), degenerative disc disease at L5-S1 (diagnosed in 2004). Her medical history also included a partial hysterectomy in 1986, sinus surgery in 1994, and a bronchoscopy procedure in 2004. She has a five-year history of smoking one pack of cigarettes daily, but quit smoking in 1982.

She reported at the first appointment that her energy was six out of ten (ten best), but her goal was ten out of ten. Her stress level was generally low and her sleep "not good." She had only been able to sleep five hours each night for the past two months due to night sweats. Sleep apnea had been ruled out per her report. She suffered from life-long post-nasal drip, was experiencing palpitations once weekly, and had an intermittent eczematous rash on her fingers bilaterally and also occasionally on her neck and abdomen. She also complained of severe brain fog, with decreased ability to process information. All other systems were negative on ROS.

Her *medications* at the time of the initial evaluation included Advair 250/50 once daily since 2004, Flonase 50 mcg once daily since 2001, HRT Bi-Est/Progesterone cream 5 mg/120 mg per gram since 2005 (but on HRT since 2000).

Physical examination revealed adventitious lung sounds in all lobes, with bronchi worse in the lower left lobe. Cardiac physical examination was normal. The patient did have slight periorbital edema and dark circles under both eyes. Her affect was generally flat, and she appeared tired.

Initial Impression and Plan: I discussed with the patient the concept that *Apergillus* infection is an opportunistic infection and that there may be things that are decreasing her immune system's ability to fight the infection. The general approach I took with her included killing the fungus while also boosting the immune system. I prescribed nebulized Fluconazole 1% (10 mg/mL) solution from a compounding pharmacy and instructed her to inhale 2 mL via a nebulizer twice daily for two months, and to take one bottle of URI Formula, a dietary supplement containing antimicrobial herbs. I discussed with her how specific nutritional deficiencies and allergies may decrease immune system function. I ordered a 1.25 hydroxyvitamin D test and a MetaCT 150 test, which contains a twenty plasma amino acid panel, a urinary organic acids panel and a ninety-food IgG allergy test.

At her follow-up on 2/14/08 we reviewed the test results (see faxed test results) and placed her on a customized treatment plan based on these results (see Treatment Plan 2/14/08).

At subsequent follow up appointments on 3/4/08 and 4/8/08, the patient reported continued improvement. Physical examination on 3/4/08 revealed all lung fields were clear to auscultation and no adventitious sounds were noted. Her first morning peak flow meter was 450, which increased from 425 per her report. Her energy, sleep, and brain fog had all improved markedly. She no longer was experiencing palpitations. At her 3/4/08 appointment she reported only coughing five to six times during the previous month, whereas she was coughing daily prior to my treating her. As of her appointment on 4/8/08, she was no longer coughing up any sputum and reported that her cough had resolved. She had discontinued the flonase and was now taking the Advair every other day instead of daily. I instructed the patient to follow up prn.

If you would like to discuss the patient's treatment, better understand the interpretation of the biochemical testing (the MetaCT 150), or discuss my general approach to pulmonary or other conditions, I would be happy to do so with you. You may also learn more by reading my book, *A Revolution in Health through Nutritional Biochemistry*, written with Steve Pieczenik, MD, PhD, or by reading the textbook I edited called, *Laboratory Evaluations for Integrative and Functional Medicine*.

Warm Regards,

John Neustadt, ND

Chapter Nineteen

Asthma

Asthma is a respiratory condition characterized decreased ability to breathe, wheezing, shortness of breath, and in severe attacks, death. This is caused by bronchoconstriction causing decreased oxygen flow. Asthma can occur in children and in adults. In children, food allergies are frequently present. Identifying these allergies with IgE and IgG Antibody test can be helpful, recommending anti-inflammatory dietary supplements to decrease inflammation in the lungs and prescribing strict avoidance of artificial colors, especially yellow dies, food additives and preservatives. In contrast, adult onset asthma, also called mature-onset asthma, occurs in adults who have no history of asthma. In adults, this condition is frequently caused by decreased production of epinephrine, a compound the body normally creates that, among other things, causes the lungs to dilate so people can breathe. The nutrients required to produce epinephrine include the amino acid tyrosine, vitamin B6, copper, and iron.

Case: Mature Onset Asthma/Pre-diabetes in a Sixty-two-year-old Male

This is the case of Dr. Pieczenik, the cofounder of NBITC. When he was sixty-two years old he presented at Montana Integrative Medicine with a previous diagnosis of mature onset, exercise-induced asthma. This condition develops in adults and results in a decreased ability to breathe during exercise or cold weather. In his case, his lungs would constrict and his pulmonologist determined that he had a 22% deficit in oxygen. He was literally short of breath all the time.

While his pulmonologist could not determine the cause of the dysfunction, he nonetheless wanted to treat it symptomatically with steroids. Steroids have been around for more than forty years, and Dr. Pieczenik could not believe that there had been no advances in medicine during that time. Steroids carry serious risk for side effects and do nothing to cure the patient; therefore, the gentleman decided to get a second opinion.

He heard of Dr. Neustadt's work in nutritional biochemistry and received a complete evaluation. His results showed that he had elevated tyrosine, low copper, a low copper-to-zinc ratio, and low epinephrine. Tyrosine flows down its pathway to form epinephrine and requires several vitamins and minerals to do so, including copper.

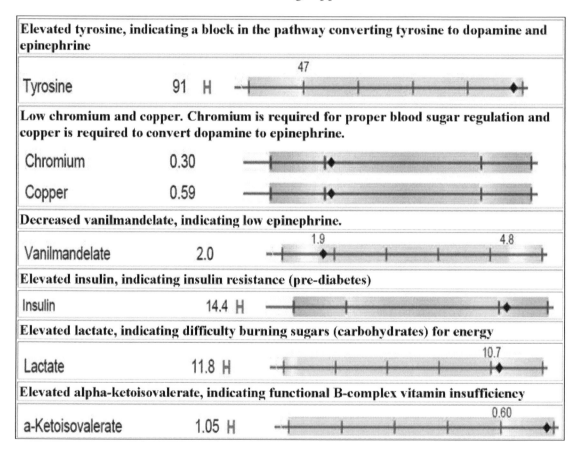

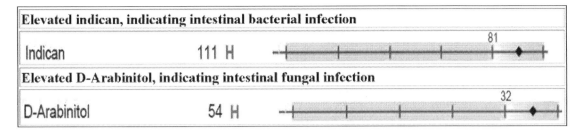

Elevated indican, indicating intestinal bacterial infection		
Indican	111 H	

Elevated D-Arabinitol, indicating intestinal fungal infection		
D-Arabinitol	54 H	

Epineprhrine is a bronchodilator, and his deficiency in epinephrine was the immediate reason why he developed mature onset asthma. The block in the pathway was at the step where dopamine is converted to norepinephrine, which requires copper. In turn, his deficiency in copper resulted from his chronic consumption of an over-the-counter dietary supplement containing high amounts of zinc without any copper in it. He was taking 50 mg of zinc daily because he had read somewhere that zinc may be helpful for his prostate; however, high amounts of zinc can decrease copper absorption. In effect, this patient induced a copper deficiency and his medical condition.

By correcting his copper, all his breathing symptoms disappeared, and upon retesting several months later, his tyrosine, copper and vanilmandelate levels had all normalized. What's important here is that the evaluation identified the underlying cause of his condition, which was treatable. His medical doctors would never even have known or understood the basic underlying functional biochemistry that led to this disorder. It was never part of their medical school education and is still not taught in conventional medical programs. Instead of merely providing steroids that at best may have only relieved the symptoms, the treatment here was to correct the underlying copper deficiency. Within two weeks of initiating the treatment plan to rebalance his biochemistry, the patient's mature onset asthma was completely resolved. He no longer requires any steroids.

Chapter Twenty

Cancer

In the United States, cancer is responsible for about 25% of all deaths each year. In the United States, breast cancer is the most prevalent cancer in women, and the second most common cause of cancer death in women (after lung cancer). In 2007, breast cancer is expected to cause 40,910 deaths (7% of cancer deaths; almost 2% of all deaths) in the United States. Women in the United States have one in eight lifetime chance of developing invasive breast cancer and a one in thirty-three chance of breast cancer causing their death. The number of cases has significantly increased since the 1970s, a phenomenon partly blamed on modern lifestyles in the Western world.

The approach to working with oncology patients using functional medicine has two purposes. First, through testing for nutritional deficiencies, it becomes possible to create customized programs for people to help build their immune system so that they can fight the cancer more effectively. This does not mean that this approach is a cure for cancer but can be viewed as an adjunct to conventional medical oncology approaches. The second is to decrease the risk of side effects from certain medications. Some chemotherapeutic drugs are known to deplete specific nutrients, which is the underlying cause of the side effects from these medications.

Surgery, radiation, and chemotherapy are frequently used alone and in combination to treat cancer. Each can be life saving, and each can cause severe side effects. Radiation can effectively kill cancerous tissue; however, radiation is nonspecific and will also damage nontarget tissues. Specifically, radiation will damage those cells that divide most rapidly, which include those lining the intestines, leading to increased risk for gastrointestinal complaints, malabsorption, and nutritional deficiencies. Chemotherapy, like many medications, causes depletions in specific nutrients. For example, Herceptin, used to treat breast cancer, can cause cardiotoxicity because it depletes L-carnitine and coenzyme Q10 (CoQ10). Testing someone's unique nutritional biochemical status and designing plans for him or her based on his or her unique needs can help speed up healing time from surgery, decrease side effects from radiation and chemotherapy, and improves someone's overall strength, sense of wellbeing, and vitality.

It's important, however, to time nutritional therapies properly in order to mitigate any risk of negative interactions with radiation and chemotherapy.

Case: Breast Cancer in a Fifty-four-year-old Woman

A fifty-four-year-old woman presented to Montana Integrative Medicine after being diagnosed with breast cancer and undergoing a radical mastectomy, radiation, and chemotherapy. She continued to be on intravenous Herceptin treatments for the cancer. She complained of severe indigestion, fatigue, insomnia, constipation, muscle aching, and spasms. She rated her energy at four out of ten, ten being best. Her nutritional biochemical test revealed multiple severe deficiencies that explained most of her symptoms.

Severe amino acid deficiencies, suggesting damage to the intestines and malabsorption			
Arginine	44 L	50 - 160	50 / 160
Histidine	62 L	70 - 140	70 / 140
Isoleucine	47 L	50 - 160	50 / 160
Leucine	72 L	90 - 200	90 / 200
Lysine	128 L	150 - 300	150 / 300
Methionine	23 L	25 - 50	25 / 50
Phenylalanine	38 L	45 - 140	45 / 140

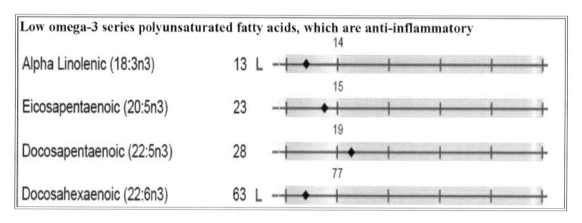

Threonine	142	100 - 250	
Tryptophan	25 L	35 - 65	
Valine	158 L	170 - 420	
Tyrosine	38 L	50 - 120	
Glutamine	397 L	600 - 1,050	
Proline	102 L	130 - 400	

Low minerals

Chromium	0.22 L	
Copper	0.48 L	
Magnesium	27 L	
Manganese	0.27	
Selenium	0.11 L	
Zinc	5.6 L	

Low omega-3 series polyunsaturated fatty acids, which are anti-inflammatory

Alpha Linolenic (18:3n3)	13 L	
Eicosapentaenoic (20:5n3)	23	
Docosapentaenoic (22:5n3)	28	
Docosahexaenoic (22:6n3)	63 L	

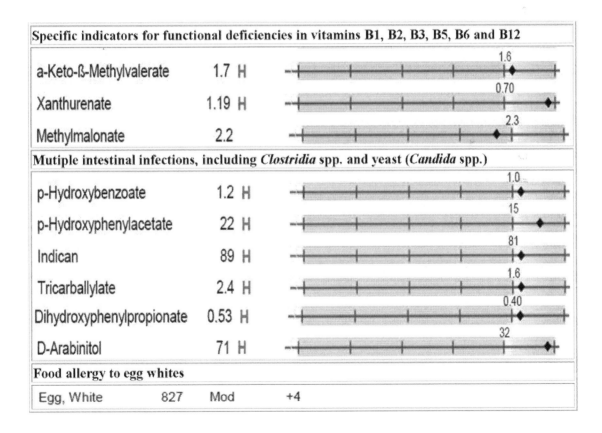

Decreased ability to burn fat for energy; functional deficiency in L-carnitine

Adipate	2.4 H	1.8
Suberate	3.4	3.4

Decreased ability to use carbohydrates for energy; functional deficiencies in vitamins B1, B3, lipoic acid and CoQ10

Pyruvate	6.8 H	4.1

Specific indicators of functional CoQ10 deficiency

Fumarate	2.71 H	0.71
Malate	4.3 H	2.3

Specific indicators for functional deficiencies in vitamins B1, B2, B3, B5, B6 and B12

a-Keto-ß-Methylvalerate	1.7 H	1.6
Xanthurenate	1.19 H	0.70
Methylmalonate	2.2	2.3

Mutiple intestinal infections, including *Clostridia* spp. and yeast (*Candida* spp.)

p-Hydroxybenzoate	1.2 H	1.0
p-Hydroxyphenylacetate	22 H	15
Indican	89 H	81
Tricarballylate	2.4 H	1.6
Dihydroxyphenylpropionate	0.53 H	0.40
D-Arabinitol	71 H	32

Food allergy to egg whites

Egg, White	827	Mod	+4

She was placed on a therapeutic program tailored specifically to her needs, which included diet and nutraceuticals. Over the next several months her muscle cramps, indigestion, and constipation completely resolved, and her energy increased to eight out of ten (ten being best). Moreover, she described a general increase in vitality and strength.

* * *

Treatment Plan

Diet:
AVOID all egg and egg products for eight weeks, then reintroduce them into your diet.

For intestinal overgrowth of yeast and bacteria:
BERBERINE FORTE: Take one capsule twice daily with food.

For low amino acids:
RESCULPT: Add two rounded scoops to a beverage of your choosing (you may add it to a smoothie, also) daily.

For low minerals:
PROMINERALS: Take three capsules daily with food. Take one bottle and then discontinue.

REJUVAMAG: Take two capsules each night before bed.

For low Vitamin D:
SUPER D: Take one capsule daily with food.

For functional vitamin deficiencies:
VITAMIN C POWDER: Mix two scoops twice daily in water, and drink with a meal.

SUPREME FEM MULTIVITAMIN (WITH IRON): Take four capsules daily with a meal.

For low iron:
FERROSOLVE: Take one capsule daily with or *without food. Note: Taking with some vitamin C can increase its absorption.*

Future treatment options:

Consider adding DIM this summer after you stop with the Herceptin therapy. DIM modulates the 2/16-hydroxy estrogen ratio. Consider L-carnitine in the future if energy doesn't increase.

Case: Large Granulomatous Leukemia in a Seventy-two year old Man

A seventy-two-year-old man drove twelve hours to seek an evaluation and treatment by Dr. Neustadt. He had a diagnosis of hypercellular marrow with T-cell lymphoproliferative disorder consistent with T-Cell Large Granular Lymphocyte Leukemia (T-LGL Leukemia) based on an iliac bone marrow aspiration and biopsy. He also had past diagnoses of insulin-dependent diabetes mellitus (IDDM) and hypertension.

At the time of his appointment he was taking the following medications: Meformin 500 mg three times daily for the past seven to eight years; Prednisone pulse starting at 40 mg daily for one week and tapering down over three weeks; Methotrexate 5 mg weekly; Metoclopramide, Co-trimoxazole (TMP/SMX), Ranitidine (Zantac), and Humulin (human recombinant insulin) as needed; Allopurinol; and Ibesartan (Karvea).

At his first appointment his chief complaints were lack of energy and weight loss. His energy was one out of ten, with ten being best. It had been that way for the previous eight months without any improvement. He had lost thirty pounds in the past three months, and weighed in at the clinic at 155 pounds. His height was 5'9.5". Not unexpectedly, physical examination revealed significant hepatosplenomegaly. The inferior border of his liver was three centimeters distal to the costal margin and the medial border of his spleen was at the midsternal line.

Multiple complete blood count reports that the patient brought with him to his first appointment showed a severe pancytopenia, with low white blood cells (WBC), red blood cells (RBC), hemoglobin, hematocrit, platelets, mean platelet volume (MPV), and neutrophils.

He elected to take the MetaCT 400 test, which revealed severe nutrient deficiencies, free radical damage, inflammation, and impaired liver metabolic pathways. He did not test positive for any food allergies, which was to be expected, since he was taking prednisone, a powerful immune suppressant.

Surprisingly, although prednisone is a strong anti-inflammatory as well, this patient tested high for c-Reactive Protein (CRP), a marker of inflammation, and two markers for free radical damage, 8-Hydroxy-2-deoxyguanosine and p-Hydroxyphenylactate (HPLA). Moreover,

8-Hydroxy-2-deoxyguanosine is a specific marker for free radical damage to DNA and has been associated with increased risk for cancer.[258]

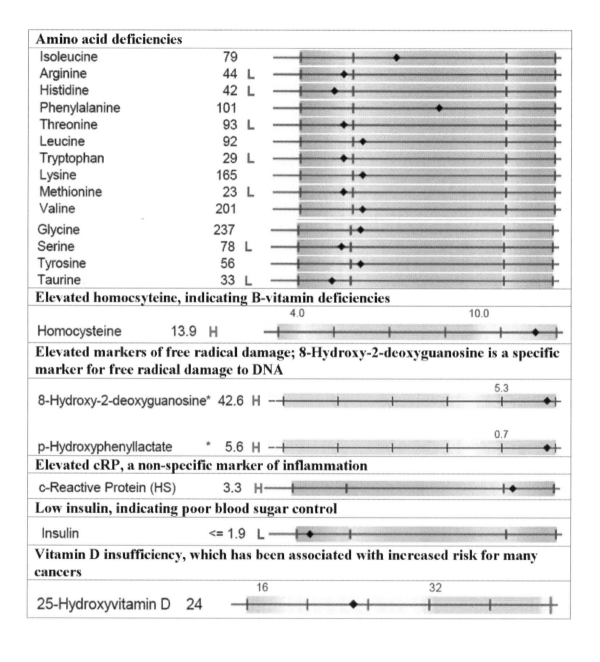

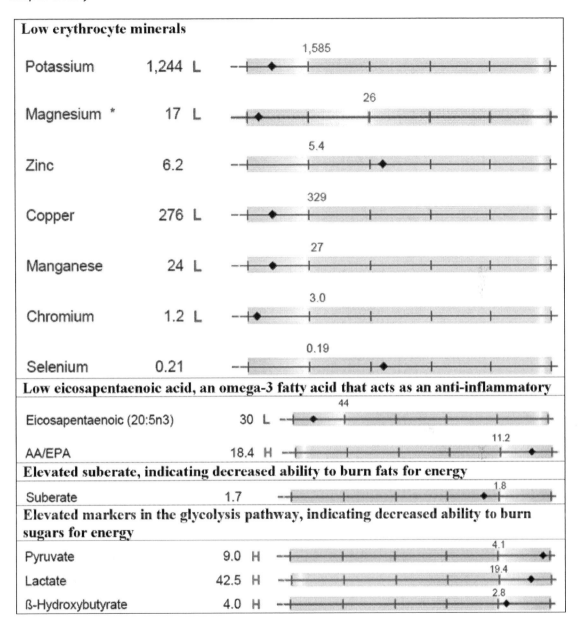

Low erythrocyte minerals

Potassium	1,244	L
Magnesium *	17	L
Zinc	6.2	
Copper	276	L
Manganese	24	L
Chromium	1.2	L
Selenium	0.21	

Low eicosapentaenoic acid, an omega-3 fatty acid that acts as an anti-inflammatory

Eicosapentaenoic (20:5n3)	30	L
AA/EPA	18.4	H

Elevated suberate, indicating decreased ability to burn fats for energy

Suberate	1.7

Elevated markers in the glycolysis pathway, indicating decreased ability to burn sugars for energy

Pyruvate	9.0	H
Lactate	42.5	H
ß-Hydroxybutyrate	4.0	H

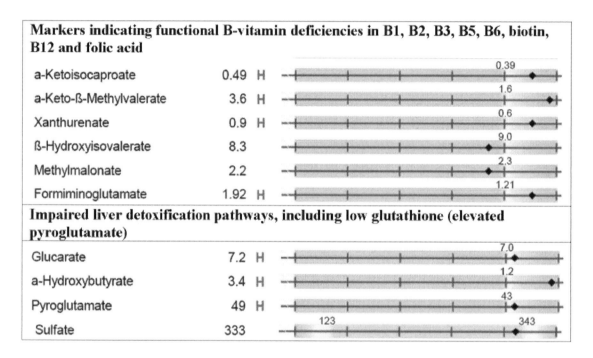

Kreb's cycle intermediates, indicating further difficulty creating cellular energy

Cis-Aconitate	74	76
Isocitrate	93 H	92
a-Ketoglutarate	26.9	27.8
Succinate	3.5	12.3
Fumarate	0.72 H	0.71
Malate	2.6 H	2.3
Hydroxymethylglutarate	9.1 H	6.8

Markers indicating functional B-vitamin deficiencies in B1, B2, B3, B5, B6, biotin, B12 and folic acid

a-Ketoisocaproate	0.49 H	0.39
a-Keto-ß-Methylvalerate	3.6 H	1.6
Xanthurenate	0.9 H	0.6
ß-Hydroxyisovalerate	8.3	9.0
Methylmalonate	2.2	2.3
Formiminoglutamate	1.92 H	1.21

Impaired liver detoxification pathways, including low glutathione (elevated pyroglutamate)

Glucarate	7.2 H	7.0
a-Hydroxybutyrate	3.4 H	1.2
Pyroglutamate	49 H	43
Sulfate	333	123 / 343

Based on this gentleman's tests, medical history, published research on leukemia and nutrition, and his symptoms, he was placed on a customized treatment plan. Over the course of several months his energy improved to eight out of ten, with ten being best, and he put on fifteen pounds. Over the course of the following year, his pancytopenia did not change; however, his quality of life while taking the presecribed nutrients remained high, with sustained energy and improved mood. Additionally, a repeat biopsy showed no progression in his bone cancer. He regained his quality of life to the point where he was able to fish and hike again, activities he had been forced to give up.

* * *

Treatment Plan

For intestinal infections:
Until such time as you discontinue your antibiotics, it is not recommended to treat the intestinal infection.

For amino acids:
CUSTOMIZED AMINO ACID BLEND: Take as directed on the bottle.

GLYCINE POWDER: Mix ½ teaspoon daily with water with or between meals. Take one bottle of this and then discontinue.

GLUTAMINE RX: Mix one teaspoon twice daily in water and drink.

TYROSINE 1g: Take one table daily.

For elevated homocysteine:
HOMOCYSTEINE FACTORS: Take one capsule twice daily with food.

For elevated lipoprotein(a) and free radical markers:
BUFFERED VITAMIN C 1,000 mg: Take three capsules daily all in divided doses.

RESVERATROL 200 mg: Take two capsules twice daily.

PROTECT DM: Take one capsule daily.

EGCG 250 mg: Take two capsules twice daily.

CURCUMIN PRO 450 mg: Take three tablets tablet three times daily.

For Coenzyme Q10 and extra magnesium:
MAG-10: Take one capsule daily with a meal.

For low vitamin D:
VITAMIN D3, 5,000 IU: Take one capsule daily with food.

For minerals:
PROMINERALS: Take three capsules daily with food. Take one bottle and then discontinue.

K+2 POTASSIUM 300 mg: Take one capsule daily with food.

For multivitamin:
SUPREME MULTIVITAMIN (WITHOUT IRON): Take four capsules daily with a meal.

For Low Omega-3 Fatty Acids:
CARLSON'S COD LIVER OIL: Take one tablespoon (equivalent of three teaspoons) daily. Keep refrigerated.

For ability to burn fats and sugars for cellular energy:
MITOFORTE: Take four capsules each morning with breakfast.

For B-vitamins:
COFACTOR B: Take one capsule daily with food.

BIOTIN 5000 MCG 60 CAPS by Allergy Research Group. Take one capsule daily.

B-12 SUBLINGUAL: Dissolve one lozenge under the tongue daily.

FA-8 FOLIC ACID 800 mcg: Take one capsule daily. Take one bottle and then discontinue.

For liver detoxification pathways:
N-ACETYL-CYSTEINE (NAC) 900 mg: Take one capsule daily with food.

For vitamin K2, which promotes bone health and has anticancer properties:
OSTEO-K 180 capsules: Take 3 capsules twice daily with meals containing some fat.

For additional support:
FRUITS N GREENS : Mix one tablespoon—approximately 6 grams—with eight ounces of water or your favorite juice *twice daily.*

Chapter Twenty-One

Chronic Pain

Pain is the most common complaint that leads patients to seek medical care. Chronic pain is not uncommon. Approximately 35% of Americans have some element of chronic pain, and approximately fifty million Americans are disabled partially or totally due to chronic pain. The definition of chronic pain is generally accepted to be pain lasting longer than six weeks, which makes this condition clinically problematic.

The burden of proof to identify the underlying cause rests with the physician. This effectively mandates that doctors order many tests, which may or may not be required. Chronic pain is one of the most difficult conditions to effectively diagnose and treat. More often than not, patients suffering from chronic pain go from doctor to doctor getting many tests ordered that don't reveal any significant information and are prescribed multiple medications to treat symptoms. However, the symptoms and frustration level of these patients just worsens. It's quite common for patients to become frustrated, demoralized, and depressed, which just compounds their problems.

To effectively treat chronic pain, one must have a very fine diagnostic tool and honed clinical skills. Fortunately, functional medicine provides the tools and clinical paradigm required to be an effective physician for these patients. Nearly 70% of the patients Dr. Neustadt sees have chronic pain as one of their complaints. This pain might be psychological, physiological, and/or structural in nature. Of those patients, almost all of them had already been to numerous other doctors and were on a minimum of four prescription medications each. These medications include analgesics, usually a non-steroidal anti-inflammatory such as Tylenol or Aleve; anti-depressants such as Prozac, Elavil (amitryptaline), Effexor (Venlafaxine); anxiolytics such as lorazapam or diazepam; and semisynthetic opiods such as hydrocodone and codeine.

What this all means is that effectively the medical profession in its attempt to merely manage symptoms is creating an iatrogenic syndrome, which increasingly requires more and more tests and more and more medications in an unrelenting spiral of ineffectiveness. This is not intentional. Patients are caught in a rigid medical model that doesn't allow for the most part for alternative perspectives, irrespective of documented outcomes.

The more appropriate paradigm for evaluating and treating chronic pain requires a more holistic approach. This includes a detailed intake that documents the attributes of pain: onset, frequency, duration, location, radiation, pain quality, pain quantity, and ameliorating and aggravating factors. However, clinicians need to not just focus on the pain the person is complaining of at the time of the appointment. A careful review of systems (ROS) will provide additional crucial information. The following are the questions Dr. Neustadt routinely asks in a ROS during an initial intake: Any fevers? Weight changes? Headaches? Visual disturbances? Post-nasal drip? Difficulty swallowing? Palpitations? Chest pain? Shortness of breath? Abdominal gas and bloating? Diarrhea or constipation? Blood or mucous in the stool? Is the urine OK—no pain on urination, frequency, urgency, nocturia, incomplete voiding, red tinge to the urine? Any joint or muscle aches or pains? Any numbness or tingling anywhere?

If any of the answers to the questions are affirmative, then Dr. Neustadt asks additional questions to identify the attributes of those symptoms and attempts to correlate them to the major patient complaint and other symptoms in the body.

There are three general categories of pain: musculoskeletal, metabolic, and infectious. The symptoms of these three categories can overlap greatly, so it's important that a skilled clinician be able to perform a complete medical history and physical exam to gather the data required to make the best clinical decision for the patient. This cannot be done in a fifteen-minute appointment, which is why the current medical model is completely unable to adequately address these problems.

In fact, physicians have a category of pain called psychogenic pain, psychophysiological pain, or psychosomatic pain. The authors believe that this label is completely condescending and primarily applied when the doctors have failed in their job of identifying the underlying causes. Instead of admitting their failure, they make the patients feel even worse by implying that the source of the pain is just all in their head and their fault. In fact, the reverse is actually true. The pain is usually quite real, and there are real, biochemical, and physiological explanations.

What's crucial in this discussion is to realize that the source of the pain is not necessarily the underlying cause of the pain. For example, food allergies and intestinal infections can cause migraine headaches, arthralgias, myalgias, and abdominal pain. Likewise, statin medications such as Lipitor can cause myalgias due to its depleting of coenzyme Q10 (CoQ10). Additionally, insomnia and anxiety can exacerbate a pain condition and hinder someone's ability to heal.

The common sources of chronic pain are damage or inflammation affecting joints (arthalgia or arthritis), muscles (myalgia or myositis), and/or nerves (neuralgia or neuropathy). Pain syndromes related to joint injury include osteoarthritis, which is the most common cause of chronic joint pain, and rheumatoid arthritis. Pain related to nerve injury includes postherpetic neuralgia, the vexing pain that may follow shingles; tic douloureux (trigeminal neuralgia), a condition that involves intense facial pain; diabetic neuropathy, which results in painful feet; and phantom limb or post-amputation pain, which may occur following the removal of a limb.

Because the organs inside the body don't have pain fibers like the joints, skin, or muscles, organ damage may be signaled by a chronic, aching, or ill-defined discomfort. This is referred to as visceral pain. Inflammation or cancer of an organ (for example, the liver, kidney, or bowel) can cause chronic visceral pain.

Chronic pain is an often debilitating condition affecting an estimated 86 million Americans. Along with unrelenting or recurrent pain, sufferers may experience depression, anxiety, and sleep disturbances. Eighty percent of chronic pain sufferers also experience depression, 63% experience irritable bowel syndrome (IBS), 80% experience allergies, and many also suffer from adrenal fatigue and intestinal dysbiosis. It's been documented that 80% of untreated, chronic pain can disrupt family life and interfere with daily functioning.

As demonstrated in multiple cases in this book, such as for migratory arthritis, abdominal pain, and headaches, functional biochemical testing and treatments can be curative. However, if the situation is due to ligament or tendon laxity, the prolotherapy may be an option. For a further discussion on prolotherapy, see the Modalities chapter. In certain cases, obviously surgery is appropriate. However, other less invasive modalities exist to help patients.

Chapter Twenty-Two

Rashes

A rash is an area of irritated or swollen skin that might be erythematous, pruritic and exhibit papules, plaques, scales, or blisters. Included in the category of rashes are all the dermatitides (e.g., atopic dermatitis, contact dermatitis, and seborrheic dermatitis), psoriasis, pityriasis, rosacea, and more. According to the Merck Manual, "Dermatitis is always the skin's way of reacting to severe dryness, scratching, an irritating substance, or an allergen."

Eighty percent of cases of contact dermatitis are caused by irritants, such as chemicals that directly damage skin. These chemicals can be acids, alkalis (such as drain cleaners), solvents (such as acetone in nail polish remover, benzene, and xylene), strong soaps, and plants (such as poinsettias and peppers). Some of these chemicals cause skin changes within a few minutes whereas others require longer exposure.

Allergic contact dermatitis is a reaction by the body's immune system to a substance contacting the skin. Sometimes a person can be sensitized by only one exposure, and other times sensitization occurs only after many exposures to a substance. After a person is sensitized, the next exposure causes itching and dermatitis within four to twenty-four hours, although some people, particularly older people, do not develop a reaction for three to four days.

Thousands of substances can result in allergic contact dermatitis. The most common include substances found in plants such as poison ivy, rubber (latex), antibiotics, fragrances, preservatives, and some metals (such as nickel and cobalt). About 10% of women are allergic to nickel, a common component of jewelry. People may use (or be exposed to) substances for years without a problem, then suddenly develop an allergic reaction. Even ointments, creams, and lotions used to treat dermatitis can cause such a reaction. People may also develop dermatitis from many of the materials they touch while at work (occupational dermatitis).

Sometimes contact dermatitis results only after a person touches certain substances and then exposes the skin to sunlight (photoallergic or phototoxic contact dermatitis). Such substances include sunscreens, aftershave lotions, certain perfumes, antibiotics, coal tar, and oils.

Atopic dermatitis is one of the most common skin diseases, affecting between 9% and 30% of children or teenagers in the United States. Almost 66% of people with the disorder develop it before age one, and 90% by age five. In half of these people, the disorder will be gone by the teenage years, whereas in others it is life long.

Doctors do not know what causes atopic dermatitis, but people who have it usually have many allergic disorders, particularly asthma, hay fever, and food allergies. The relationship between the dermatitis and these disorders is not clear because atopic dermatitis is not an allergy to a particular substance. Atopic dermatitis is not contagious.

Many conditions can make atopic dermatitis worse, including emotional stress, changes in temperature or humidity, bacterial skin infections, and contact with irritating clothing (especially wool). In some infants, food allergies may provoke atopic dermatitis.

There are many other types of rashes, and a complete discussion of them here is beyond the scope of this book. The points the authors simply want to illustrate are that there are many causes of rashes and that the underlying causes of many rashes, especially atopic dermatitis, are unknown. If underlying causes, such as exposure to an environmental toxin, as in the case of contact dermatitis, are at fault, then eliminating the exposure is key to the treatment.

Dr. Pieczenik

Clearly most rashes are seen by dermatologists. In a simplistic fashion Dr. Pieczenik was taught in medical school the following principles. If it's wet, dry it; and if it's dry, wet it. And for the rest, put steroids on it. That is a simplistic approach; but, nonetheless, it encompasses the basic truths of treating dermatological disorder. Obviously if an infection is involved physicians treat with antibiotics or antifungals. If it is cancer then patients may go through a very sophisticated procedure, called a Mohs' Procedure, especially for basal cell carcinoma. In this procedure the patient is being treated by a board-certified dermatologist and surgeon who evaluates the skin biopsies at the time of the surgery and determines if they should surgically remove more tissue or if they've cut out enough and have removed the entire cancer.

They have had quite impressive outcomes with this procedure because it's a real-time evaluation without experiencing the usual delay between excision and receipt of the pathology report. In this case the dermatologist is also the surgeon and the pathologist especially trained in both of these skills. So, in effect, dermatology today ranges from the most simplistic descriptive diagnostic criteria and treatments (e.g., steroids, methotrexate, enbrel, which is simply a sophisticated and extremely expensive anti-inflammatory medication) to the highly specialized surgical interventions. However, the number of specialists trained in the Mohs' Procedure is very limited, and so most patients will not have access to this potentially life-saving medicine.

One key point is that these treatments, except surgical excision of cancer and the identification and removal of an irritant in contact dermatitis, are symptomatic and not curative.

Dr. Neustadt

Naturopathic, or Functional, Dermatology really boils down to two simple ideas: (1) identify and remove the cause and (2) enhance the body's natural detoxification pathways to remove any toxins from the body. In doing so, Dr. Neustadt and other physicians who practice functional medicine may evaluate for food allergies, intestinal infections, and optimal functioning of liver metabolic pathways. As discussed in the chapter, "Heal the Gut, Heal the Body," food allergies can cause rashes and joint pain. The following cases detail how this approach can be used successfully to treat rashes.

Case: Migratory Rash in a Fifty-four-year-old Woman

A fifty-four-year-old woman made an appointment in the fall of 2007 with Dr. Neustadt. She had been suffering for one year with a rash. The woman owned several different apartments with her husband, and they would do the maintenance on the properties themselves. One of their apartments had been abandoned by the tenants, and when they entered the property to clean it out, they noticed strong chemical smells. There appeared to be chemical stains on the walls and on the carpets, as well as mounds of trash in the apartment. The patient stated that she thought the apartment may have been used to manufacture drugs. She and her husband spent the entire day cleaning the apartment. That night when she went home a rash started on her face. In the coming weeks the rash would come and go several times a week, and her face and lips would be so swollen that she felt embarrassed to even be seen in public.

The rash initially started on the right aspect of her tongue with edema and dysphagia. It improved with Benadryl. The rash was migratory and moved all over her body. It would last from twenty-four hours to three days before resolving in any given location. The rash exhibited no pain, discharge, scabbing, or flaking. She would occasionally experience bruising at the site of the rash, and the rashes were pruritic. She tried taking Zyrtec, which had been prescribed to her by a local allergist, without relief. She had been seeing this allergist for eleven months. He had prescribed prednisone, to which the patient experienced an adverse event, which she described as feeling "drunk" on the medicine. The prednisone was discontinued.

Review of system was all essentially normal except for her report of the rash. Her stress level overall was low. Her sleep was "really good," and she awoke refreshed each morning. She also rated her energy as "good," at an eight out of ten, with ten being best.

Physical examination revealed an overweight woman with a BMI of 27.7 and with elevated blood pressure of 140/94. However, the patient reported that the day before the physical examination her blood pressure was 128/84. Skin evaluation showed two areas of rash approximately 2x2 inches located a couple of inches below each breast. These rashes were erythematous patches without discharge.

A MetaCT 150 test was ordered to evaluate for liver detoxification pathways and general nutritional status. This panel evaluates for 90 different IgG food allergies, 20 plasma amino acids and urinary organic acids for functional nutritional deficiencies. This panel is a good baseline test for most patients.

Inability to burn fat for energy, explaining her difficulty losing weight		
Adipate	6.0 H	5.7
Suberate	1.1	1.8
Ethylmalonate	7.0 H	5.5

Decreased Kreb's Cycle Intermediates leading to inefficient ATP production

Analyte	Value		Reference
Citrate	894		948
Cis-Aconitate	78	H	76
Isocitrate	91		92
a-Ketoglutarate	36.3	H	27.8
Succinate	11.2		12.3
Fumarate	0.93	H	0.71
Malate	2.1		2.3

Functional B-vitamin deficiencies (B1, B3, B5, B6, biotin)

Analyte	Value		Reference
a-Ketoisocaproate	0.46	H	0.39
Xanthurenate	0.9	H	0.6
ß-Hydroxyisovalerate	12.5	H	9.0

Elevated marker of inflammation

Analyte	Value		Reference
Quinolinate	13.7	H	10.2

Elevated detoxification pathway analytes, indicating compromised ability to metabolize toxins; 2-Methylhippurate, in particular, indicates xylene exposure and elevated pyroglutamate indicates glutathione deficiency.

Analyte	Value		Reference
2-Methylhippurate	0.067	H	0.050
Orotate	0.4		1.0
Glucarate	6.1		7.0
a-Hydroxybutyrate	0.4		1.2
Pyroglutamate	152	H	60
Sulfate	362		166 390

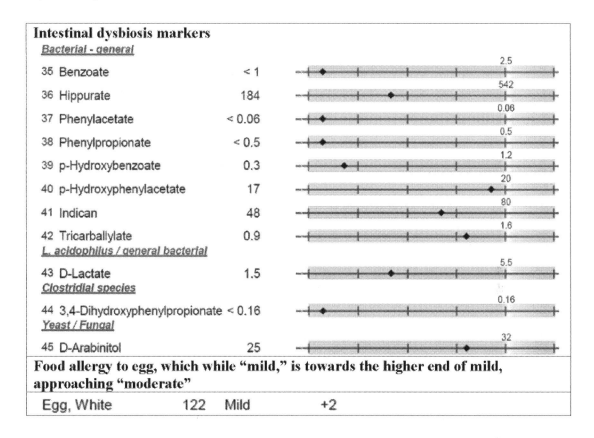

Intestinal dysbiosis markers		
Bacterial - general		
35 Benzoate	< 1	
36 Hippurate	184	
37 Phenylacetate	< 0.06	
38 Phenylpropionate	< 0.5	
39 p-Hydroxybenzoate	0.3	
40 p-Hydroxyphenylacetate	17	
41 Indican	48	
42 Tricarballylate	0.9	
L. acidophilus / general bacterial		
43 D-Lactate	1.5	
Clostridial species		
44 3,4-Dihydroxyphenylpropionate	< 0.16	
Yeast / Fungal		
45 D-Arabinitol	25	

Food allergy to egg, which while "mild," is towards the higher end of mild, approaching "moderate"

Egg, White	122	Mild	+2

At her two-week follow up, the patient reported being compliant with all of the recommendations on the treatment plan (below). Since starting the plan she had been having daily outbreaks of the rash. She reported purchasing a face mask with a filter to wear while working at her properties, and using a HEPA filter at home. At her six-week follow up appointment she reported that she had lost two pant sizes on the treatment plan and was very excited about it. She went from a size fourteen to a size twelve pant. She continued to be compliant with the treatment plan and reported that she had not had any rashes in the prior three weeks. Physical examination revealed no rashes. She reiterated at that time the rashes were occurring daily before starting the plan.

At her twelve-week follow up after initiating the plan she reported that she had only had three rashes in the prior six weeks since her last appointment. She continued to take her Zyrtec. Five months later the patient returned and reported that she was having a rash outbreak every two weeks, but that the severity of the rash had decreased by more than 80% and the duration of the rash at each outbreak decreased by approximately 99%, according the patient. Before starting the treatment plant the rash would last two to three days and as of this follow up appointment the rash would only last a "few hours," according to the patient. This approach resulted in decreasing the severity, frequency, and duration of the rash to the point where the rash became only a minor inconvenience to the patient and was no longer debilitating. This was accomplished without any steroids or pharmaceuticals.

* * *

Treatment Plan

Diet:
AVOID all *eggs and egg products* for eight weeks, and then reintroduce them into your diet.

Lifestyle:
Purchase a face mask with filter to use while working on your properties and a HEPA filter to use at home.

For intestinal dysbiosis:
BERBERINE FORTE: Take one capsule twice daily with food.

ENTEROPRO: Take one capsule daily with food. Keep refrigerated.

For amino acid deficiencies:
Note: You may combine the amino acid powders and take them at the same time.

RESCULPT: Stir or blend two scoops (23g) of ReSculpt into 8 fl. oz. of water, milk, or juice once daily.

GLYCINE POWDER: Mix ½ teaspoon daily with water with or between meals. Take one bottle of this and then discontinue. This recommendation is based on elevated 2-Methylhippurate (indicating exposure to xylene.

Here's some information about xylene:

2-Methylhippurate is a by-product from the detoxification of the common solvent, xylene. Xylene is oxidised via the hepatic P450 oxidase enzymes and then conjugated with glycine during Phase II detoxification. Xylene can be found in new paint, paint thinners, building products, fuel and exhaust fumes, dry cleaning fluid, new cars, new carpets, industrial degreasers and solvents. Accumulation of toxins such as xylene can result in increased oxidative stress.

For vitamins and minerals:

SUPREME MULTIVITAMIN (WITHOUT IRON): Take four capsules daily with a meal.

MITOFORTE: Take four capsules each morning with breakfast.

COFACTOR B: Take one capsule daily with food.

MAG-10: Take one capsule daily with a meal.

BIOTIN 5000 MCG: Take one capsule daily.

FA-8 FOLIC ACID 800 mcg: Take one capsule daily. Take one bottle and then discontinue.

B-12 SUBLINGUAL: Dissolve one lozenge under the tongue daily. Take one bottle and then discontinue.

For inflammation:

CURCUMIN PRO: Take two tablets twice daily for one month, then one tablet twice daily thereafter.

PROTECT DM: Take one capsule daily.

Chapter Twenty-Three

Migraine Headaches

Migraine headaches can cause debilitating pain so severe that relief is only obtained by lying down in a dark, quiet place. Migraines afflict twenty-eight million Americans, with females suffering more frequently (17%) than males (6%). The pain usually is on one side of the head, although about a third of the time the pain is on both sides. People suffering from migraines may also experience nausea, vomiting, diarrhea, cold hands, cold feet, and sensitivity to both light and sound. Typically, attacks can last from four to seventy-two hours.

Many different contributing factors have been implicated in the etiology of migraine headaches. There is little doubt that food allergy/intolerance plays a role in many cases of migraine headache. Many double-blind, placebo-controlled studies have demonstrated that the detection and removal of allergic foods will eliminate or greatly reduce migraine symptoms in the majority of patients. Identifying and eliminating food allergies resulted in success ranges from 30 to 93%, with the majority of studies showing a remarkably high degree of success.[259-263]

Low erythrocyte magnesium has been associated with migraine headaches. In a study of 152 migraine cases and eighty-five controls, erythrocyte magnesium determinations was 2.04 mmol/litre in migraine patients and 2.32 mmol/litre in controls ($P < .0005$).[264] In all migraine cases in this study, without exception, clinical evaluation showed an abnormal sensitivity of the buccofacial and cervical muscles which was unilateral and homolateral when migraine was unilateral; it was bilateral when migraine was bilateral. The muscles which were the most sensitive to palpation were the sternocleidomastoid, external pterygoid, and scalene. These findings show that migraine patients have a magnesium deficit, which, while not constant, is a frequent occurrence.

This raises the problem of the relationship between migraine and other disorders characterized by magnesium deficit, such as latent tetany, mitral valve prolapse, and certain allergies. This magnesium deficit probably promotes muscle irritability, especially when a local imbalance factor results in a permanent pathological stimulation. In addition to irritation and hypersensitivity, migraine attacks occur, particularly after stress and digestive, endocrine, and neurological problems.

In a double-blind, placebo-controlled trial at the University Centre for Adaptive Disorders and Headache (UCADH) in Italy, twenty women suffering with menstrual migraine were given 360 mg/day of Mg or placebo on the fifteenth day of the cycle and continued till the next menses, for two months.[265] The Pain Total Index (PTI) significantly decreased in the treatment group compared to controls ($P < .03$) and the number of days with headache was reduced only in the patients on active drug. Magnesium also improved premenstrual complaints, which, along with the PTI score, continued to be reduced at the fourth month of treatment when magnesium was supplemented in all the volunteers. Intracellular magnesium levels in patients with menstrual migraine were reduced compared to controls, which was increased during. An inverse correlation between PTI and intracellular polymorphonuclear (PMN) magnesium content was demonstrated. These data point to magnesium supplementation as a further means for menstrual migraine prophylaxis, and support the possibility that a lower migraine threshold could be related to magnesium deficiency.

Other deficiencies, such as in vitamin B2 (riboflavin), have also been described as a possible hypothesis for migraines. The potential mechanism relates to mitochondrial dysfunction, concomitant reduction of energy production and cerebral blood vessels instability. If this hypothesis is true, riboflavin, which has the potential of increasing mitochondrial energy efficiency, might have preventive effects against migraine. To test this hypothesis, forty-nine patients suffering from migraine were treated with a very large dose (400 mg daily) of riboflavin for at least three months.[266] Overall improvement after therapy was 68.2% in the riboflavin group as determined by the migraine severity score used in the study. No side-effects were reported. The results from this preliminary study suggest high-dose riboflavin could be an effective, low-cost preventive treatment of migraine.

Noteworthy here is the connection between mitochondrial damage and migraine headaches. This connection has been noted elsewhere.[267] Unfortunately, all the clinical trials to date have adopted a pharmacological model of evaluating a monotherapy (e.g., magnesium or riboflavin) for a condition that is essentially multifactorial. When speaking about mitochondrial damage, there are many nutrients, including vitamins, minerals, amino acids and antioxidants that are required for proper mitochondrial function. These include iron, sulfur, vitamin B1 (thiamin), riboflavin, vitamin B3 (niacin), vitamin B6 (pantothenic acid), cysteine, magnesium, manganese, lipoic acid, copper, zinc, l-carnitine, vitamin C and ubiquinone (Coenzyme Q10).[267-269]

Case: Migraine Headache and Depression in a Twenty-three-year-old Woman

A twenty-three-year-old woman had been suffering for seven years with migraine headaches. Up until one year prior to seeing Dr. Neustadt, she had been getting migraine headaches three times each year; however, the frequency had increased, and at her first appointment at Montana Integrative Medicine she complained of suffering debilitating daily migraine headaches. Her migraines were accompanied by visual disturbances that manifested as seeing "little stars all over" and pain. A careful medical history revealed that her migraine headaches began when she was in high school and suffering from anorexia nervosa and intense periods of exercise. She had also been experiencing depression and fatigue. Given her medical history and chief complaint of migraine headaches, she was at high risk for underlying nutritional deficiencies.

When she was evaluated by Dr. Neustadt, she was taking three different medications for migraine headaches, Relpax, Zanaflex, and Ultracet, and one antidepressant medication, Fluoxetine (Prozac). This woman also suffered from painful periods (dysmenorrhea), for which she would have to take Tylenol. One day prior to each period, she would become so emotional that she would break down in tears, and she stated that her mood was quite erratic.

Her biochemical testing revealed the underlying causes for her symptoms. She had severe amino acid deficiencies; food allergies; functional deficiencies in B-complex vitamins, of which the most severe was vitamin B6; functional deficiency in carnitine (elevated adipate), meaning that she was having difficulty burning her fats for cellular energy; liver detoxification pathway impairment (elevated orotate); and food allergies to dairy and eggs.

Food allergies (IgG 90-Antigen test)

Casein	324	Mod	+3
Chicken	< 10		
Egg, White	157	Mod	+3
Egg, Yolk	15		
Lamb	< 10		
Milk	406	Mod	+3

Amino acid deficiencies

Amino acid	Value		Marker
Arginine	50	L	56
Histidine	65		63
Isoleucine	30	L	43
Leucine	67	L	81
Lysine	106	L	124
Methionine	15	L	17
Phenylalanine	44	L	47
Threonine	70	L	79
Tryptophan	35	L	38
Valine	112	L	154
Serine	66	L	71
Taurine	35		33
Tyrosine	39	L	42

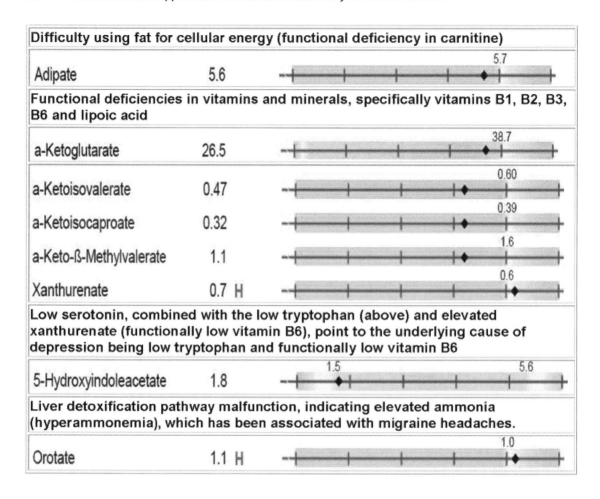

She was placed on a therapeutic diet and specific nutrients to replete her deficiencies. After two weeks on her therapeutic diet and nutraceuticals, she reported a 60% improvement in the intensity of her migraine headaches. Additionally, whereas she was experiencing migraines daily before, she had only experienced one migraine in the previous two weeks. She could resume her daily activities without any interference from the migraines, and the flashes of light had also improved. With respect to her mood, she stated that her mood was "a lot better; more stable," and her premenstrual syndrome had completely resolved.

After being on the program for six weeks, she continued to experience improvements in her symptoms. She had only experienced one migraine in the month since her previous appointment, and that was after traveling and eating foods to which she was allergic. She also stated her depression had completely resolved and requested that Dr. Neustadt begin weaning her off her antidepressant medications. After twelve weeks she reported no migraine headaches, no PMS and that her mood was "excellent."

Case: Migraine Headaches in a Thirty-six-year-old Woman

A thirty-six-year-old woman made an appointment with Dr. Neustadt complaining of migraine headaches. She would only experience migraine headaches occasionally but had had them twice since the birth of her daughter, seventeen months ago. She also complained of fatigue, with her energy being five out of ten, with ten being best; post-nasal drip every day for more than a year, which had been treated with multiple rounds of antibiotics; and difficulty losing weight. Prior to the pregnancy with her daughter, her energy was nine out of ten. She had a history of gestational diabetes and hyperemesis gravidum for seven months during her pregnancy with her daughter.

Her MetaCT 150 test revealed:

Decreased ability to burn fats for energy		
Adipate	7.4 H	6.0
Suberate	3.2 H	1.9
Ethylmalonate	1.6	2.0
Decreased ability to burn sugars for energy*		
Pyruvate	3.4 H	3.3
L-Lactate	13	14
Elevated malate, a Kreb's Cycler intermediate that is a sensitive indicator of functional CoQ10 deficiency		
Malate	3.1 H	1.5
Functional deficiencies of B-complex (B1, B2, B3, B5), biotin and B12		
a-Keto-ß-Methylvalerate	0.96 H	0.69
ß-Hydroxyisovalerate	5.9 H	4.7
Methylmalonate	1.2	1.3
Low 5-Hydroxyindoleacetate, a marker of serotonin catabolism		
5-Hydroxyindoleacetate	1.5 L	1.6 ... 8.1

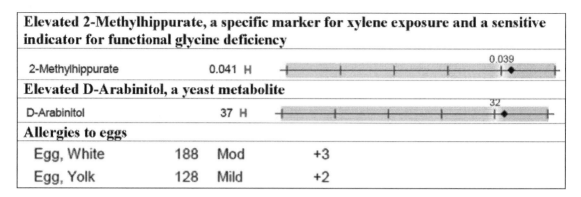

Elevated 2-Methylhippurate, a specific marker for xylene exposure and a sensitive indicator for functional glycine deficiency			
2-Methylhippurate	0.041 H		0.039
Elevated D-Arabinitol, a yeast metabolite			
D-Arabinitol	37 H		32
Allergies to eggs			
Egg, White	188	Mod	+3
Egg, Yolk	128	Mild	+2

*Note: A fasting blood sugar test ordered through the local hospital showed high-normal fasting blood sugar, with a reading of 105 mg/dL (70–110). After being on the treatment plan for six weeks, her fasting blood sugar was retested and it was 94 mg/dL. This drop in fasting blood sugar correlated with her improvement in symptoms.

She was placed on a customized treatment plan (below) for three months. After being on the plan for six weeks she reported that her pants were fitting looser, her energy had increased, her post-nasal drip had resolved, and her migraine headaches also had resolved. The patient's symptoms all continued to improve throughout the program.

* * *

Treatment Plan

Diet:
AVOID all *eggs and egg-containing products* for eight weeks, and then reintroduce them into your diet.

For fungal overgrowth (dysbiosis):
Rx NYSTATIN TABLETS, 500,000 units twice daily for three months.

BERBERINE FORTE: Take one capsule twice daily with food. Take four bottles of this and then discontinue.

ENTEROPRO: Take one capsule daily with food. Keep refrigerated.

For ability to burn fat and sugars for energy:

MITOFORTE: Take four capsules each morning with breakfast.

MAG-10: Take one capsule daily with a meal.

For B-complex vitamins:

COFACTOR B: Take one capsule daily with food.

BIOTIN 5000 MCG: Take one capsule daily.

B-12 SUBLINGUAL: Dissolve one lozenge under the tongue daily.

Additional vitamin and mineral support:

SUPREME FEM MULTIVITAMIN (WITH IRON): Take four capsules daily with a meal.

REJUVAMAG: Take two capsules each night before bed.

For liver detoxification:

GLYCINE POWDER: Mix ½ teaspoon daily with water with or between meals. Take one bottle of this and then discontinue.

LIVER SUPPORT: Take two capsules twice daily. Take one bottle and then discontinue.

For amino acids:

GLUTAMINE RX: Mix one teaspoon twice daily in water and drink.

Chapter Twenty-Four

Seizure Disorder

Epilepsy is a disorder characterized by the occurrence of at least two unprovoked seizures twenty-four hours apart. Some clinicians are also diagnosing epilepsy when one unprovoked seizure occurs in the setting of an interictal discharge. Seizures are the manifestation of abnormal hypersynchronous discharges of cortical neurons. The clinical signs or symptoms of seizures depend on the location of the epileptic discharges in the cortex and the extent and pattern of the propagation of the epileptic discharge in the brain.

Seizures are a common, nonspecific manifestation of neurologic injury and disease. This should not be surprising because the main function of the brain is the transmission of electrical impulses. The lifetime likelihood of experiencing at least one epileptic seizure is about 9%, and the lifetime likelihood of receiving a diagnosis of epilepsy is almost 3%. However, the prevalence of active epilepsy is only about 0.8%.

There are many types of seizures that have been described, including tonic-clonic seizures, absence seizures, pseudo-seizures, shuddering attacks, and status epilepticus. Regarding morbidity, trauma is not uncommon among people with generalized tonic-clonic seizures. Injuries such as ecchymosis; abrasions; and tongue, facial, and limb lacerations often develop as a result of the repeated tonic-clonic movements. Atonic seizures are also frequently associated with facial and neck injuries. Worldwide, burns are the most common serious injury associated with epileptic seizures.

Regarding mortality, seizures cause death in a small proportion of individuals. Most deaths are accidental due to impaired consciousness. However, sudden unexpected death in epilepsy (SUDEP) may occur even when patients are resting in a protected environment (e.g., in a bed with rail guards).

The goal of treatment is to achieve a seizure-free status without adverse effects. Many different medications exist that affect specific neurotransmitters, such as gamma-amino butyric acid (GABA) as with phenobarbital, benzodiazepines; sodium channel blockers such as phenytoin, carbamazepine, and oxcarbazepine; glutamate (an excitatory amino acid) modulators, such as topiramate, lamotrigine, felbamate; calcium channel blockers, such as ethosuximide, lamotrigine, and valproate; and carbonic anhydrase inhibitors, such as topiramate and zonisamide.

Dr. Pieczenik

In most cases the conventional medical approach to diagnosis and treatment of seizures is consistently effective. The diagnostic categories are so finite in their difference that only specialists (i.e., neurologists) would know the differences. Mapping of neural networks, electrical conductivity studies, and computational analysis of how the brain works has given researchers and clinicians the ability to understand the brain's basic biochemical and physiological dynamics better than ever before. They are now able to tie it appropriately to psychiatric, behavioral and neurological disorders.

The origins of psychiatry lie in neuropsychiatry, and the ability to connect organic disorders such as primary seizure disorders with biochemical determinants makes neurology a partner with psychiatry. This is the one area in medicine where causality, and not just symptoms, have propelled this field into other disciplines, such as immunology, pathology, computational biology, and molecular biology. In effect, Dr. Pieczenik predicts that neurology and psychiatry will merge, coming back together as one discipline, just as it was approximately one hundred years ago. He thinks that it's important to remember that Sigmund Freud, the father of psychoanalysis, which has had a major influence on psychiatry in the last fifty years, was a neurologist and not a psychiatrist.

Dr. Neustadt

Several cases of seizure disorders have been worked up by Dr. Neustadt. It is important to note that of those three (one partial seizure disorder in a child, one gran mal seizure in an adult, and one pseudo-seizure disorder in an adult) only the gentleman with pseudo-seizure disorder was directly helped by this approach. The patient's neurologist had tried every seizure and antidepressant medication on this patient, and yet the seizures and depression continued without any improvement. This was truly a case where conventional medicine had tried its best and failed, not because of any incompetence, but simply because of the limits of knowledge in neurology and psychiatry.

The premise of this case was that the low-normal homovanillate, the marker for dopamine, was low, thereby causing the seizures, similar to the tremors that occur in Parkinson's disease. In fact, when the patient was evaluated by Dr. Neustadt, the doctor observed tremors in the patient that reminded Dr. Neustadt of Parkinson's disease. This begs the question as to whether Carbidopa/Levadopa would have helped this patient's seizures. Instead of pursuing a pharmacological approach, Dr. Neustadt instead identified the specific nutritional deficiencies contributing to the low homovanillate and subsequently provided those nutrients. The seizures resolved.

Can the successful outcomes of this case be repeated in other patients? Dr. Neustadt is not sure. However, the results were so spectacular, and continued for over two years of follow-up that this approach deserves more inclusive study from different perspectives. The doctor who referred this patient to Dr. Neustadt said, "This man was so desperate that without Dr. Neustadt's intervention, the patient would have died."

Case: Pseudo-seizures in a Thirty-seven-year-old Man

A thirty-seven-year-old male presented with seizures, life-long depression, suicidal tendencies, and extreme fatigue. This was a man who was literally at death's doorstep—he was exhausted, unable to care for himself, and without hope. His seizures had begun four months earlier while on a pleasure trip to Las Vegas. He had no history of head trauma or previous seizure activity. He was evaluated by a neurologist who ordered a computer tomography (CT) scan, a magnetic resonance imaging (MRI) study, and an electroencephalogram (EEG). All of these studies were appropriate for the medical model, and all would have been ordered by Dr. Neustadt;

however, the crucial difference between the nutritional biochemistry approach and that of a well-educated conventional neurologist is that Dr. Neustadt also ordered a comprehensive nutritional biochemistry evaluation.

All conventional imaging ordered by the neurologist revealed no abnormalities. The patient was diagnosed as having "pseudo-seizures" (literally, "false seizures"), yet there was nothing false about them. The patient was prescribed different anti-seizure medications, but none reduced his seizure symptoms at all. Instead, he developed increasing depression because he felt more and more helpless and hopeless because none of his symptoms were relieved after seeing these medical experts.

When he finally arrived at Montana Integrative Medicine and took the comprehensive nutritional biochemistry test, his results explained the underlying causes all of his symptoms. His depression was a result of low epinephrine, low serotonin, low omega-3 fatty acids, and a functional vitamin B6 deficiency. His seizures were due to low phenylalanine, low tyrosine, low dopamine, and functionally low vitamin B6, which is required for dopamine formation. Low dopamine causes seizures and is an underlying cause of Parkinson's disease. Additionally, his medical evaluation, which included a diet recall, made it apparent that the timing of his seizures appeared to coincide with possible low blood sugar, which is documented to cause seizures.

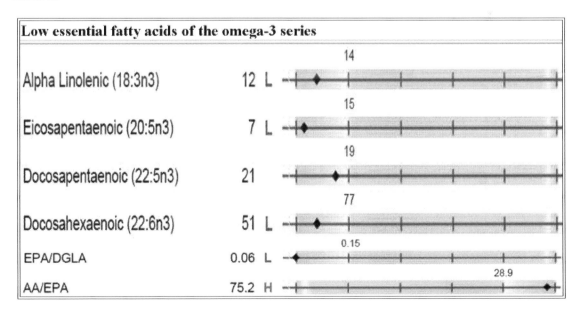

Amino acid imbalances; specifically, low glycine, an inhibitory neurotransmitter; and low-normal phenylalanine and tyrosine, the prescursors to dopamine.

Phenylalanine	55	45 - 140	
Glycine	171 L	225 - 450	
Serine	68 L	90 - 210	
Taurine	52	50 - 250	
Tyrosine	60	50 - 120	
Gamma-Aminobutyric Acid	6.6 H	<= 5.0	

Functional vitamin B6 deficiency

Xanthurenate	0.70	

Neurotransmitter imbalances, with low homovanillate (marker for dopamine)

Vanilmandelate	1.6 L	
Homovanillate	1.1 L	
5-Hydroxyindoleacetate	2.0	

Low-normal minerals

Chromium	0.29	
Manganese	0.26	

He was placed on a comprehensive treatment plan that included nutritional cofactors to correct his underlying biochemical dysfunction and a medically-directed diet to better control his blood sugar. He was prescribed amino acids, high-dose B-vitamins, essential fatty acids, a high-quality multivitamin and mineral supplement, and a high-fiber diet. The patient's seizures stopped after being on the program for four days, and he continued to be seizure-free at the three-month follow up appointment. He also reported no more depression, increased energy, no suicidal thoughts, and feeling better than he could ever remember.

* * *

Treatment Plan

Diet:

AVOID *all milk, milk products, and anything that contains casein* for eight weeks, and then reintroduce them into your diet.

For low amino acids:

RESCULPT: Stir or blend two scoops (23g) of ReSculpt into 8 fl. oz. of water, milk, or juice once daily.

GLUTAMINE RX: Mix one teaspoon twice daily in water and drink.

GLYCINE POWDER: Mix ½ teaspoon twice daily with water.

TAURINE POWDER: Take 1/2 teaspoon daily on an empty stomach (thirty minutes before eating or 1.5 hours after eating).

For vitamin and mineral deficiencies:

SUPREME MULTIVITAMIN (WITHOUT IRON): Take four capsules daily with a meal.

VITAMIN C POWDER: Mix two scoops twice daily in water, and drink with a meal.

SUPER D3: Take one capsule daily with food.

CARLSON'S COD LIVER OIL: Take one tablespoon (equivalent of three teaspoons) daily.

COFACTOR B: Take one capsule daily with food.

MAG-10: Take one capsule daily with a meal.

N-ACETYL-CYSTEINE (NAC) 1,000 mg: Take one capsule daily with food.

Appendix A

Modalities

The authors decided to include a chapter on different modalities in clinical practice for several reasons. First, these are the primary modalities Dr. Neustadt learned through his formal naturopathic medical training, and they are what he applies successfully to various patient problems every day. Ironically, Dr. Pieczenik had a vague familiarity with these modalities because his father, Dr. Saul Pieczenik, used many of these modalities in his private practice from the 1950s through the 1960s in Harlem, New York. Dr. Pieczenik's father was a French-trained physician who was taught about nutritional medicine, prolotherapy, hydrotherapy, and other modalities. Interestingly, Dr. Saul Pieczenik, who was a medical doctor, essentially received what is today the naturopathic medical curriculum.

In contrast, Dr. Steve Pieczenik received the classical American conventional medical education from Cornell University Medical College and Harvard Medical College, both excellent schools. However, neither in his formal education nor in his subsequent career in medicine and psychiatry did he ever hear of any references whatsoever to any of these modalities. The first time Dr. Steve Pieczenik ever heard of nutritional medicine was his encounter with Dr. Neustadt in 2005. It is important to understand that naturopathic medicine, or any of these modalities, were never denigrated in Dr. Pieczenik's formal education; they were simply never mentioned. It's as if naturopathic physicians, nutrional medicine, the clinical application of biochemistry to patient problems, functional testing, and prolotherapy simply did not exist. And still does not exist.

The ***only*** modalities that Dr. Pieczenik was taught were the classical modalities of drugs and surgery, and almost zero prevention. His journey to this point is a function of having met Dr. Neustadt and the vague reflections of his father's shadow. As a boy, Dr. Pieczenik remembers his father administering prolotherapy, B-vitamin shots, and diathermy to patients. And people got better. In fact, Dr. Pieczenik's father was one of the founders of the Health Insurance Plan (HIP) in New York, the first health maintenance organization in the country in the late 1940s.

Nutritional Medicine

Nutritional medicine is the application of concepts in nutrition to clinical medicine. This and our previous two books, *A Revolution in Health through Nutritional Biochemistry* and *A Revolution in Health Part 2: How to Take Charge of Your Health* provide the overall concepts of nutrional medicine and how clinicians and the lay public can apply them. Diet and lifestyle are the foundation of health, and the careful application of medical nutrition is a powerful and life-saving modality. It's imperative that every physician at least understands, if not accepts, this reality.

A review of the clinical trials into the use of nutrients reveals that the vast majority of adverse effects are minor and temporary. Whereas medications more often than not carry the risk of dangerous side effects, dietary supplements usually carry the risk of *side benefits,* which is a term the authors created to describe the potential indirect benefits to using nutrients in addition the direct benefits that are being targeted clinically.

A striking illustration of side benefits involved a sixty-year-old Vietnam veteran who was suffering from extreme fatigue and photophobia (sensitivity to light). When he awoke in the morning, his energy would be good, but he had to nap every three hours during the day because his energy would diminish to nothing. While in the clinic, he requested the window shades be drawn because of his extreme sensitivity to light. Biochemical testing revealed several abnormalities in his energy-producing pathways, amino-acid deficiencies, free-radical damage to his DNA (a risk factor for cancer), problems with his liver-detoxification pathways, and an intestinal bacterial infection. His major complaint was extreme fatigue, and the treatment plan was tailored to correct his biochemical abnormalities to provide more energy. One month later, he returned and only had to nap once a day. To his surprise, his light sensitivity had also greatly improved. The window blinds did not have to be drawn, and his wife reported that he had enough energy to start riding his motorcycle again.

The problem is that many people who object to using nutrients clinically are simply unfamiliar with the basic research and clinical trials supporting its use. The National Institute of Health (NIH) manages the nation's largest database of peer-reviewed scholarly journals, which can be accessed at www.pubmed.com. There are more than six million entries in its database, which is a phenomenal amount of research. A search for all studies on the amino acid carnitine yields more than nine thousand entries and a search for vitamin C returns over twelve thousand entries. It is the authors' assertion that those who state that research does not support the use of nutrients in clinical practice have simply not done their homework.

Most physicians and people in the general public do not know even the most basic concepts in nutritional medicine. One of the things the authors would like to begin teaching people is how they can evaluate the quality of a dietary supplement formulation. This will ensure that the person is getting their money's worth, but also that they aren't taking nutrients or combinations of nutrients that may actually harm them. For example, Dr. Pieczenik unwittingly took high amounts of zinc without balancing it with copper and induced a copper deficiency, which created his asthma. The following frequently asked questions will hopefully help demystify dietary supplement labels for readers and keep them safe and healthy.

What Are Dietary Supplements?

Dietary supplements are vitamins, minerals, herbs, and other substances meant to improve your health. They can come as pills, capsules, powders, and liquids. It's important to realize that they are not intended to replace an optimal diet, but rather to "supplement" the diet.

Dietary supplements are regulated by the U.S. Food and Drug Administration (FDA) under the Dietary Supplement Health and Education Act of 1994 (DSHEA). Signed by President Clinton on October 25, 1994, the DSHEA acknowledges that millions of consumers believe dietary supplements may help to augment daily diets and provide health benefits.

The provisions of DSHEA define dietary supplements as being:

- A product (other than tobacco) that is intended to supplement the diet that bears or contains one or more of the following dietary ingredients: a vitamin, a mineral, an herb or other botanical, an amino acid, a dietary substance for use by man to supplement the diet by increasing the total daily intake, or a concentrate, metabolite, constituent, extract, or combinations of these ingredients.
- Intended for ingestion in pill, capsule, tablet, or liquid form.
- Not represented for use as a conventional food or as the sole item of a meal or diet.
- Labeled as a "dietary supplement."
- Products such as an approved new drug, certified antibiotic, or licensed biologic that was marketed as a dietary supplement or food before approval, certification, or license (unless the Secretary of Health and Human Services waives this provision).

Should I Take Dietary Supplements?

Most people would probably benefit from a high-quality dietary supplement. This is because most people do not eat an optimal diet. A good dietary supplement is a smart insurance policy. Basically, what a good regimen of dietary supplements, diet, and exercise do is to boost your immune system and prevent acute and chronic diseases, including heart disease, diabetes, high blood pressure, dementia, and Parkinson's disease. In medicine nutrients are even used to treat many diseases; however, patients must seek out a skilled doctor knowledgeable in nutritional medicine, since conventional physicians are not trained in nutrition.

In theory, we should be able to receive all the nutrition we need from diet alone. But the fact is that most of us do not.

- Few of us eat the recommended five to eight servings of fresh fruits and vegetables a day.
- Our food is often picked before it is ripe and transported long distances.
- The soil in which our food is grown has become depleted of nutrients.
- We rely on quick, processed foods with our busy lifestyle.
- We live in a highly toxic world.
- We have individual health needs and challenges.

A multiple vitamin and mineral (MVM) supplement does not replace a good diet. There are compounds in food that just can't be replaced in a pill. Evidence shows that a good diet is still your best tool for staying healthy. However, a good MVM supplement is important insurance for optimal health.

How Do I Know if a Dietary Supplement Is Good?

There are three things to look for in evaluating a dietary supplement. First, it should be manufactured at an *FDA-approved facility that is also GMP-certified*. Manufacturers cannot advertise this on their product labels, so you'll need to check their sales literature for this. This process requires manufacturers test raw materials for contaminants and quarantine the materials throughout the manufacturing process.

Second, the best dietary supplements will also be tested for *purity and potency*. This costs companies extra money, so they want to advertise this on their dietary supplements. Look for "tested for purity and potency" or "purity and potency guaranteed" on the labels. If they are tested for purity and potency, then the company should have on file a *certificate of analysis* for each product. A certificate of analysis verifies the purity and potency of a product. You have the right to request copies of certificates of analysis from dietary supplement companies. If they refuse to provide this to you then the product may have

Table 25.1 Quality Checklist

☑ Capsules (not tablets)
☑ More than "one-a-day" multivitamin
☑ Purity and Potency Guaranteed
☑ FDA-Approved, GMP-certified Manufacturer
☑ Highly bioavailable forms (no "-oxide" minerals)
☑ Hypoallergenic
☑ Avoid "other ingredients" (e.g., binders and fillers)

contaminants such as toxic metals, bacteria, and fungal spores in it. Additionally, you cannot be guaranteed that what's on the label is actually what's in each capsule or tablet. In fact, many studies have shown that many dietary supplements contain toxic metals and do not have the amount of nutrients in the capsules or tablets that are listed on the bottle.

Third, when discussing dietary supplements Dr. Neustadt is fond of saying, "the devil's in the details." In addition to the two requirements mentioned above, when evaluating a multivitamin and mineral supplement you should look for three things on the label. One is to check if it's a *tablet versus a capsule*. Tablets are generally more difficult to break apart in your stomach and may pass through your body without actually being dissolved and without you absorbing the nutrients. Additionally, companies tend to put poorly absorbable forms of nutrients in their formula. (More on this in a few sentences.) Next, *is it a one-a-day multivitamin?* If it is, then you're pretty much guaranteed that it's a tablet and that the nutrients it contains are of exceedingly poor quality. How can you verify this?

The last thing to do is look on the supplement facts label. This is where each ingredient is listed out in detail. Look for just three things: magnesium, zinc, and copper. *If any minerals are in an "oxide" form, then the product is garbage.* This is because these minerals are very poorly absorbed in their "oxide" form. For example you can only absorb about 2% of the magnesium as magnesium oxide. This means that 98% of what you put in your mouth is just passing right through you and being eliminated in your stool. In fact, magnesium oxide is so poorly absorbed that it's used in higher amounts as a laxative! Companies use the oxide form of minerals because their *very* inexpensive. But you'd be better off eating a few spinach leaves than wasting your money on a dietary supplement that contains minerals in their oxide forms. See Table 25.1 for a dietary supplement checklist.

The bottom line is that it truly is a situation of *buyer beware*. The consumer needs to become educated and proactive to ensure they're getting their money's worth, but also to protect themselves from poisoning from toxic metals and other contaminants. A 2006 survey of Ayurvedic dietary supplements produced in South Asia and sold in 20 stores in the Boston area revealed that 20% of the dietary supplements (14 of 70 Ayurvedic supplements) contained heavy metals.[270] Of those with heavy metals, 13 contained lead at median concentration of 40 µg/g (5–37,000 µg/g), 6 tested positive for arsenic at median concentration of 430 µg/g (37–8,130 µg/g), and 6 contained mercury at median concentration of 20,225 µg/g (28–104,000 µg/g). The EPA established reference doses (RfDs) for oral chronic exposure of arsenic and mercury is 0.3 µg/kg per day,[270] which calculates to 15 µg per day for a 50 kg person. No safe level of lead consumption has been established by the U.S. Environmental Protection Agency (EPA), but levels are set by the U.S. Food and Drug Administration (FDA).

An earlier 2002 case report documented lead poisoning from Ayurvedic medicine in a 41year-old male.[271] He complained of malaise, weakness, abdominal pain, and weight loss. His blood lead level was 78 µg/dL and it was anemic (hemoglobin 7.9 g/dL). He had traveled to India where he was treated with Ayurvedic medicine for oligospermia (decreased sperm number). Analysis of the dietary supplements revealed high concentrations of lead—13,084 µg/g in one pill and 1,917 µg/g in another pill. It was estimated that during the course of his treatment he had ingested 1.26 g of lead.

Another 2002 case report described arsenic toxicity in a 39 year-old woman taking the dietary supplement Chitosan,[272] derived from chitin, a polysaccharide found in shellfish. Chitosan is believed to help people lose weight by blocking the absorption and storage of fat. The woman reported to the emergency room complaining of fatigue, headache, and weakness for the past 6 months. She had been taking 6 capsules daily of the "fat blocker" pills for a year. A 24-hour urine collection revealed 186 µg/L arsenic (nl: 0–50 µg/L). Analysis of the pills revealed an arsenic concentration of 135.5 ng/g/capsule. Shellfish is a known reservoir of arsenic, and no other sources could be identified.

A meta-analysis of 22 case reports, case series, and epidemiological research concluded, "heavy metal (particularly lead) poisoning through traditional Chinese medicine use has been reported with some regularity."[273]

What Are Bioavailable Forms of Nutrients?

Bioavailable Forms

There are better forms of individual nutrients than others. You get what you pay for. Many lower cost products will use cheaper forms of vitamins and minerals. Unfortunately, many times cheaper forms also mean nutrients which are poorly absorbed or not usable by the body. Below are a few examples of nutrient choices.

- *Vitamin E*

  The best form of Vitamin E is d-alpha tocopherol with mixed tocopherols (d-alpha, gamma, beta, and delta). The synthetic form of Vitamin E is dl-alpha tocopherol. Note that the difference in labeling is "d" vs. "dl" before the alpha—"dl" is not a healthy choice.

- *Vitamin B12*

  The best form of Vitamin B12 is methylcobalamin. Cyanocobalamin is the form in most vitamins and is usually fine for most people. If someone has chronic disease, however, a methylcobalamin form is recommended.

- *Vitamin B6*

  The active form of B6 is pyridoxine 5-phosphate. This is usually designated at P-5-P.

- *Minerals*

  There are many forms of minerals which are bonded to compounds; the physical form of a mineral is usually designated by the last word of the name. Example: magnesium *citrate* or magnesium *oxide*. Each form has different amounts of the basic elemental mineral as compared to the size of the whole compound and will determine how absorbable the mineral is.

For example: calcium carbonate (this includes coral calcium) is a large molecule with a lot of elemental calcium. The large size of this molecule means that it is not easily absorbed. Calcium carbonate also tends to be constipating for some people. Calcium citrate, by contrast, is a smaller form of elemental calcium, and is much more easily absorbed than the carbonate form. (An interesting note is that certain antacid medications contain calcium carbonate and are marketed as a source of calcium. However, because the purpose of an antacid is to inhibit stomach acid, and stomach acid is necessary for making minerals available for absorption, the body has a harder time actually utilizing the calcium!)

Similarly, magnesium oxide is poorly absorbed and causes water to stay in the intestines, thus causing a looser stool. Thus, magnesium oxide can be useful to treat occasional constipation. Alternatively, magnesium citrate is a better choice because it is more easily absorbed. (Caution, however, the citrate form may also cause loose stools for some people.)

There are other forms of mineral compound chelates including gluconate, aspartate, asparotate, and lactate. The gluconate form is not recommended.

What Does Hypoallergenic Mean?

A good dietary supplement will be *hypoallergenic*, meaning it does not contain wheat, dairy, soy, or artificial dyes or colorings.

What Are "Other Ingredients"?

Before you read what the active ingredients are, read the label for "other ingredients." Many supplements contain extra ingredients that may cause side effects or impair absorption. If you have lots of unnecessary "other ingredients," it does not matter how much active ingredients you have, the MVM supplement is already a poor choice. We recommend researching any ingredient that is unfamiliar to you.

The following is *not* a comprehensive list. Some "other ingredients" to avoid:

- *Glucose, fructose, dextrose, maltodextrose, corn syrup, sucrose, lactose.* These are sugars and unless these are added for flavor in children's chewable vitamins, they are not needed. As soon as possible, wean your child from a chewable to a capsule to minimize their dependence on sugar and risk to their teeth.
- *Sorbitol.* This is a sugar alcohol, and although is not purely sugar, it is not beneficial in a vitamin. For diabetics this is an absolute must for avoidance! Sorbitol can also cause diarrhea.
- *NutraSweet, Equal, Aspartame, Sucralose, Splenda.* These are artificial sweeteners and are *not* beneficial to the body.
- *Polyethylene glycol.* Although non-toxic, this chemical, when used in large dosages, is a treatment for constipation. It is unnecessary for use in highly absorbable vitamins.
- *Mineral Oil.* Mineral oil is derived from petroleum and prevents absorption of nutrients. Given these two facts, taking a vitamin with mineral oil does not seem a good choice.
- *Canuba Wax.* Canuba wax may inhibit the digestion of the ingredients and make it less absorbable. This is especially true if digestive weaknesses are already present.
- *Dextrin.* This is a binding product, making the nutrients less available for digestion.
- *Di-calcium phosphate.* Di-calcium phosphate is an excipient (an inactive ingredient) and is not available to the body as calcium. A vitamin labeling both calcium and phosphorus may be counting the di-calicum phosphate as calcium, but it really doesn't add much to the calcium content nutritionally.
- Any *coloring*
- Any *pharmaceutical glaze*

What Does GMP Mean?

GMP refers to the Good Manufacturing Practice Regulations promulgated by the U.S. Food and Drug Administration (FDA) under the authority of the Federal Food, Drug, and Cosmetic Act. These regulations require manufacturers take steps to ensure that their products are safe, pure, and effective. GMP regulations require a quality approach to manufacturing, enabling companies to minimize or eliminate instances of contamination, mixups and errors. This in turn protects the consumer from purchasing a product that is not effective or even dangerous.

Failure of firms to comply with GMP regulations can result in very serious consequences, including recall, seizure, fines, and jail time. GMP regulations address issues including recordkeeping, personnel qualifications, sanitation, cleanliness, equipment verification, process validation, and complaint handling.

Are There Any Potentially Toxic Nutrients?

While most nutrients in dietary supplements do not appear to have any toxic side effects, there are some notable exceptions. For example, very high doses of vitamin B6 (pyridoxine), a water soluble vitamin, can cause numbness and tingling in your fingers and arms. This side effect is generally reversible when you discontinue the vitamin B6. Similarly, high doses of vitamin B3 (niacin) can cause flushing ("hot flashes") and liver damage.

The amount of nutrients in dietary supplements are by and large too low to cause any problems, but sometimes people take very high amounts of nutrients because they read or heard somewhere that they may be helpful. We caution people against doing this without first discussing it with a health care provider who is an expert in nutritional medicine. Table 25.2 lists nutrients and their potential toxicities.

Table 25.2. Nutritents and their potential toxicities

Nutrient	Toxic Dosage	Symptoms and Diseases
Biotin	n/a	No side effects from oral administration at therapeutic doses have been reported
Boron	>10 mg	No side effects reported
Calcium	>2,000 mg	Drowsiness, extreme lethargy, impaired absorption of iron, zinc, and manganese, calcium deposits in tissues throughout body, mimicking cancer on X-ray
Carotene	>300 mg	Orange discoloration of skin, weakness, low blood pressure, weight loss, low white cell count
Chromium	>50 mg	Dermatitis, intestinal ulcers, kidney and liver impairment

Copper	15 mg	Fatigue, poor memory, depression, insomnia, increased production of free radicals, may suppress immune function. Violent vomiting and diarrhea. Cooking acid foods in unlined copper pots can lead to toxic accumulation of copper.
Fluoride, acute	500 mg	Poisons several enzymes, (5,000 mg lethal)
Fluoride, chronic	5 mg	Fluorosis (white patches on teeth), bone abnormalities
Folic acid	15 mg	Abdominal distention, loss of appetite, nausea, sleep disturbances, may interfere with zinc absorption, may prevent recognition of vitamin B12 deficiency
Iodine	2 mg	Thyroid impairment, iodine poisoning, or sensitivity reaction
Iron	Variable	Intestinal upset, interferes with zinc and copper absorption, loss of appetite, not safe for those with iron storage disorders such as hemosiderosis, idiopathic hemochromatosis, or thalassemias. Toxic build-up in liver, pancreas, and heart
Magnesium	N/A	Diarrhea at large dosages of poorly absorbed forms (like Epsom salts). Disturbed nervous system function because the calcium-to-magnesium ratio is unbalanced; catharsis, hazard to persons with poor kidney function.
Manganese	75 mg	Toxicity only reported in those working in manganese mines or drinking from contaminated water supplies, which results in loss of appetite, neurological damage, loss of memory, hallucinations, hyperirritability, elevation of blood pressure, liver damage. Mask-like facial expression, blurred speech, involuntary laughing, spastic gait, hand tremors.
Niacin (B3), acute	100 mg	Transient flushing, headache, cramps, nausea, vomiting
Niacin (B3), chronic	3 gm	Anorexia, abnormal glucose tolerance, gastric ulceration, elevated liver enzymes. Excessive uric acid in blood, possibly leading to gout. See Thiamin.

Pantothenic acid (B5)	High dose	Occasional diarrhea. Increased need for thiamin, possibly causing thiamin deficiency symptoms.
Phosphorous	High dose	Distortion of calcium-to-phosphorus ratio, creating relative deficiency of calcium.
Potassium	High dose	Mental impairment, weakness. Excessive potassium in blood, causing muscular paralysis and abnormal heart rhythms.
Pyridoxine (B6)	300 mg	Sensory and motor impairment. Dependency on high doses, leading to deficiency symptoms when one returns to normal amounts.
Riboflavin (B2)	N/A	No toxic effects have been noted. See Thiamin.
Selenium	750 mcg	Diabetes, garlic-breath odor, immune impairment, loss of hair and nails, irritability, pallor, skin lesions, tooth decay, nausea, weakness, yellowish skin
Thiamin (B1)	N/A	No toxic effects noted for humans after oral administration. However, since B Vitamins are interdependent, excess of one may produce deficiency of others.
Vitamin A, acute (infant)*	75,000 IU	Anorexia, bulging fontanelles, hyperirritability, vomiting
Vitamin A, acute (adult)*	2 million IU	Headache, drowsiness, nausea, vomiting
Vitamin A, chronic (infant)*	10,000 IU	Premature epiphyseal bone closing, long bone growth retardation
Vitamin A, chronic (adult)*	50,000 IU	Anorexia, headache, bluffed vision, loss of hair, bleeding lips, cracking and peeling skin, muscular stiffness and pain, severe liver enlargement and damage, anemia, fetal abnormalities (pregnant women must be very careful), menstrual irregularities, extreme fatigue, liver damage, injury to brain and nervous system.
Vitamin B12 (Cobalamin)	N/A	No side effects from oral administration have been reported. (See thiamin)

Vitamin C, acute	10 gm	Nausea, diarrhea, flatulence
Vitamin C, chronic	3 gm	Increased urinary oxalate and uric acid levels in rare cases, impaired carotene utilization, chelation (binding of vitamin C with minerals) and resultant loss of minerals may occur, sudden discontinuation can cause rebound scurvy. Kidney and bladder stones, urinary tract irritation, increased tendency for blood to clot, breakdown of red blood cells in persons with certain common genetic disorders (such as glucose-6-phosphate dehydrogenase deficiency, common in persons of African origin), may induce B12 deficiency.
Vitamin D, acute	70,000 IU	Loss of appetite, nausea, vomiting, diarrhea, headache, excessive urination, excessive thirst
Vitamin D, chronic	10,000 IU	Weight loss, pallor, constipation, fever, hypocalcaemia. In infants, calcium deposits in kidneys and excessive calcium in blood; in adults, calcium deposits throughout the body (may be mistaken for cancer) (pregnant women must be careful), deafness, nausea, kidney stones, fragile bones, high blood pressure, high blood cholesterol, increased lead absorption.
Vitamin E	1,000 IU	The safe dose is probably over 2,000, but some people experience weakness, fatigue, exacerbation of hypertension, increased activity of anticoagulants at 1,000 IU.
Vitamin K		No known toxicity with natural vitamin K (vitamin K1 and K2). Synthetic vitamin K (vitamin K3) can be toxic.
Zinc	75 mg	Gastrointestinal irritation, vomiting, adverse changes in HDL/LDL cholesterol ratios, impaired immunity. Nausea, anemia, bleeding in stomach, premature birth and stillbirth, abdominal pain, fever. Can aggravate marginal copper deficiency. May produce atherosclerosis.

*Note: Most multivitamin formulas do not contain vitamin A. Rather they contain beta-carotene, which the body converts to vitamin A. Dietary supplement labels will say, Vitamin

A (as Beta Carotene). There is no toxicity associated with taking beta-carotene, since the body will only convert as much beta-carotene to vitamin A that it needs.

Should Any Nutrients Be Balanced with Other Nutrients?

Yes. Frequently dietary supplement manufacturers will combine nutrients in ways that are potentially harmful. In other cases they don't even include nutrients that should be there to protect someone from toxicity. For example, zinc and copper must be balanced in about a ten-to-one ratio or serious disease can result. That is, for every 10 mg of zinc you need about 1 mg of copper. This is because high amounts of zinc that are not balanced with copper can cause a copper deficiency. This can result in anemia, fatigue, and breathing difficulties. This is exactly what happened to Dr. Pieczenik. He was taking zinc because he read that it could boost his immune system. But the store-bought dietary supplements with high zinc did not contain any copper. This led to a copper deficiency, which was identified by laboratory analysis, an inability to produce epinephrine, which allows the lung to dilate for breathing, and adult onset asthma. Once his copper deficiency was corrected, he no longer had asthma.

Are There Contaminants in Dietary Supplements?

Unfortunately, yes. Many studies have been published recently documenting toxic contaminants in dietary supplements. Toxic metals identified in dietary supplements include lead, arsenic, and mercury at extremely high doses. All of these toxic metals were contained in dietary supplements with raw materials from China. That is why NBI does not use any ingredients from China. Other contaminants found in dietary supplements include pesticides, dangerous fungal spores, bacteria, hormone and even some drugs. To ensure the safety of all its products, NBI pays extra to have every batch of its dietary supplements *independently tested for authenticity, potency, heavy metals, solvent residue, herbicide and pesticide residue, aflatoxins, stability, and bacteria, yeast, and mold counts.* If your dietary supplement manufacturer does not do this, you may very well be putting your health at risk.

Are All NBI Dietary Supplements High Quality?

Yes. All NBI dietary supplements conform to the highest quality manufacturing guidelines and are guaranteed for purity and potency. They have only the most absorbable nutrients in them, are hypoallergenic and do not contain any binders or fillers. They are also based on clinical trials and basic research.

Botanical Medicine

What Is Botanical Medicine?

Botanical medicine, also called herbal medicine or phytomedicine, refers to the use of any plant's seeds, berries, roots, leaves, bark, or flowers for medicinal purposes. The oldest medical systems in the world extensively used plants as medicine. In fact, the majority of the world's population to this day still turns to botanical medicines before they reach for pharmaceuticals. Throughout the ages, humans have relied on nature to supply the materials they need for their basic needs—for the production of foodstuffs, shelters, clothing, means of transportation, fertilizers, flavors, fragrances, and medicines.

Plants have formed the basis of sophisticated traditional medical systems that have been in existence for thousands of years and continue to provide the world with new remedies. Botanical medicine is based on empirical findings over thousands of years, and although some of the therapeutic properties attributed to plants have been proven false, modern clinical research supports the use of plant medicines more often than not.

Recently, the World Health Organization estimated that 80% of people worldwide rely on herbal medicines for some aspect of their primary health care. In the last twenty years in the United States, increasing public dissatisfaction with the cost of prescription medications, combined with an interest in returning to natural or organic remedies, has led to an increase in the use of herbal medicines. In Germany, roughly six hundred to seven hundred plant-based medicines are available and are prescribed by approximately 70% of German physicians.

The first records of botanical medicines, written on clay tablets in cuneiform, are from Mesopotamia and date from about 2600 BC; among the substances that were used were oils of *Cedrus* species (cedar) and *Cupressus sempervirens* (cypress), *Glycyrrhiza glabra* (licorice), *Commiphora* species (myrrh), and *Papaver somniferum* (poppy juice), all of which are still used today for the treatment of ailments ranging from coughs and colds to parasitic infections and inflammation.[274]

The rise of the pharmaceutical industry in the United States did not begin until the twentieth century. The industry started during World War I and really took off after World

War II. The premise of pharmaceutical companies' business model is that through the use of chemical processes, which in themselves are toxic, drugs can be created from natural products by isolating and concentrating specific elements of those natural substances. Using the isolated chemical or chemicals from plants and fungi, they can then cure diseases by literally providing a drug for the symptoms themselves. For example, antidepressant medications merely alleviate the symptoms of depression but do not cure depression.

How Do Herbs Work?

For most herbs, the specific ingredient that causes a therapeutic effect is not known. Whole herbs contain many ingredients, and it is likely that they work together to produce the desired medicinal effect. Many factors affect how effective an herb will be. For example, the type of environment (climate, bugs, soil quality) in which a plant grew will affect its components, as will how and when it was harvested and processed.

How Are Herbs Used?

For the reasons described in the previous section, herbalists prefer using whole plants rather than extracting single components from them. Whole plant extracts have many components. These components work together to produce therapeutic effects and also to lessen the chances of side effects from any one component. Several herbs are often used together to enhance effectiveness and synergistic actions and to reduce toxicity. Herbalists must take many things into account when prescribing herbs. For example, the species and variety of the plant, the plant's habitat, how it was stored and processed, and whether or not there are contaminants.

What Is Herbal Medicine Good For?

Botanicals are used to treat many conditions, such as asthma, eczema, premenstrual syndrome, rheumatoid arthritis, migraine, menopausal symptoms, chronic fatigue, and irritable bowel syndrome, among others. Herbal preparations are best taken under the guidance of a trained professional. Be sure to consult with your doctor or an herbalist before self-treating. Some common herbs and their uses are discussed below. Please see our monographs on individual herbs for detailed descriptions of uses as well as risks, side effects, and potential interactions.

- **Ginkgo (*Ginkgo biloba*)**, particularly a standardized extract known as EGb 761, appears to produce improvements in awareness, judgment, and social function in people with Alzheimer's disease and dementia. In a year-long study of 309 people with Alzheimer's disease, those taking EGb 761 consistently improved while those on placebo worsened.

- **Kava kava (*Piper methysticum*)** has become popular as a treatment for anxiety, but recent reports have traced liver damage to enough people who have used kava that the U.S. FDA has issued a warning regarding its use and other countries, such as Germany and Canada, have taken kava off of the market.

- **St. John's wort (*Hypericum perforatum*)** is well known for its antidepressant effects, and an analysis of twenty-seven studies involving more than two thousand people confirmed that the herb is an effective treatment for mild to moderate depression.

- **Valerian (*Valeriana officinalis*)** has had a long tradition as a sleep-inducing agent, with the added benefit of producing no hangover feeling the next day.

- **Echinacea preparations (from *Echinacea purpurea* and other Echinacea species)** may bolster immunity. In a study of 160 volunteers with flu-like symptoms, echinacea extract reduced both the frequency and severity of cold symptoms.

Is There Anything I Should Watch Out For?

Used correctly, many herbs are considered safer than conventional medications, but botanicals sourced from India and China can have toxic amounts of lead, arsenic, and other heavy metals. Therefore, readers should only purchase dietary supplements that contain herbal ingredients from companies that test the raw materials for contaminants. If it doesn't say "purity and potency guaranteed" on the bottle, and readers are uncertain if a particular manufacturer tests for contaminants, then contact the manufacturer directly. They should be willing to tell you. If they are not, then do not purchase their products.

Additionally, some botanicals, such as St. John's wort, can interfere with medications. Consult a health care provider who is an expert in herb-drug interactions before taking any dietary supplements if you are also taking any medications. Finally, some botanicals can induce abortions in women and pass into the breast milk. Therefore, women who are pregnant or nursing should only take herbal products after consulting a knowledgeable health care provider.

Nature Cure

Nature cure is a constructive method of treatment which aims at removing the basic cause of disease through the rational use of the elements freely available in nature. It is not only a system of healing, but also a way of life, in tune with the internal vital forces or natural elements comprising the human body. It is a complete revolution in the art and science of living.

Although the term "naturopathy" is of relatively recent origin, the philosophical basis and several of the methods of nature cure treatments are ancient. It was practiced in ancient Egypt, Greece, and Rome. Hippocrates, the father of medicine (460–357 B.C.) strongly advocated it. India, it appears, was much further advanced in older days in natural healing system than other countries of the world. There are references in India's ancient sacred books about the extensive use of nature's excellent healing agents such as air, earth, water, and sun. The Great Baths of the Indus Valley civilization as discovered at Mohenjodaro in old Sind testifies to the use of water for curative purposes in ancient India.

The modern methods of nature cure originated in Germany in 1822, when Vincent Priessnitz established the first hydropathic establishment there. With his great success in water cure, the idea of drugless healing spread throughout the civilized world and many medical practitioners throughout the civilized world and many medical practitioners from America and other countries became his enthusiastic students and disciples. These students subsequently enlarged and developed the various methods of natural healing in their own way. The whole mass of knowledge was later collected under one name, Naturopathy. The credit for the name Naturopathy goes to Dr. Benedict Lust (1872–1945), and hence he is called the Father of Naturopathy.

Nature cure is based on the realization that man is born healthy and strong and that he can stay as such as living in accordance with the laws of nature. Even if born with some inherited affliction, the individual can eliminate it by putting to the best use the natural agents of healing. Fresh air, sunshine, a proper diet, exercise, scientific relaxation, constructive thinking, and the right mental attitude, along with prayer and meditation, all play their part in keeping a sound mind in a sound body.

Prolotherapy

Musculoskeletal pain can be debilitating. Whether it's pain in the knees, low back, neck wrists, or ankles, everyone experiences this discomfort at some time in their lives. It's been estimated that over their lifetimes, 80% of Americans suffer from low back pain. There are many potential reasons for musculoskeletal pain. It can be from tight muscles, from direct injury from sports or a car accident, and even from food allergies or infections. But the most commonly overlooked cause of musculoskeletal pain is ligament or tendon instability.

Ligaments are bands of connective tissue that connect two or more bones. Tendons are bands of connective tissue that connect muscles to bone. Both of these structures—ligaments and tendons—are frequently damaged just by normal wear and tear. There are a lot of nerves at the spots where the ligaments and tendons attach to bones. When the ligaments and tendons are weakened, additional stress can be placed on these attachments and cause pain. George Hackett, MD, one of the founders of the techniques and education in prolotherapy in the United States concluded that up to 90% of people have degenerative changes in their weight bearing joints (low back, hips, knees, etc.) by the age of forty.

There are many causes for pain, and an integrative pain specialist will conduct a thorough interview with the patient and a detailed physical exam. Many pain treatments just suppress the symptoms with anti-inflammatories (e.g., Aleve, Ibuprofen, Tylenol) and steroids. However, if the underlying cause is ligament or tendon instability, then in most cases it can be corrected with prolotherapy. The pain is relieved and function is restored.

Prolotherapy is a simple, natural technique. It has been used and studied for more than seventy years. Usually all that's injected is a simple solution contain dextrose, glucosamine, some vitamin B12, and a local anesthetic.

The underlying cause of musculoskeletal pain is often a weakened ligament. Prolotherapy can restore joint integrity and relieve pain from:

- *arthritis*

- *whiplash*

- *sciatica*

- *disk problems*

- *low back pain*

- *rotator cuff (shoulder) pain*

- *tennis elbow*

- *old sports injuries that are now acting up*

- *knee pain (osteoarthritis, ACL or PCL injuries)*

- *TMJ (temporomandibular joint) dysfunction.*

Prolotherapy works by exactly the same process that the human body naturally uses to stimulate the body's healing system, a process called inflammation. The technique involves the injection of a proliferant (a mild irritant solution) that causes an inflammatory response which "turns on" the healing process. The growth of new ligament and tendon tissue is then stimulated. The ligaments and tendons produced after Prolotherapy appear much the same as normal tissues, except that they are thicker, stronger, and contain fibers of varying thickness, testifying to the new and ongoing creation of tissue. *The ligament and tendon tissue which forms as a result of Prolotherapy is thicker and stronger than normal tissue, up to 40% stronger in some cases!*

The concept of strengthening ligaments goes back to the time of Hippocrates. Reports of shoulder joint instability and its many repair methods date back to Hippocrates' treatise, "On Joints." Hippocrates described the practice of using cautery to cause the capsule to scar and thus tighten around the joint. While his technique is no longer used, the underlying concept is similar to Prolotherapy—strengthen the ligaments.

In the 1930s many case reports emerged in France and the United States of musculoskeletal disorders, such as TMJ, knee pain, and sacroiliac joint (SI joint, which holds your pelvis to your lower back), being successfully treated with Prolotherapy. In 1956, George Hackett, MD, a surgeon, published the first edition of the textbook *Ligament and Tendon Relaxation Treated by Prolotherapy.* Dr. Hackett reported a twelve-year success rate of 82% in the treatment of eighteen hundred patients with back pain using Prolotherapy.

Then, in 1983, microscopic examination of rabbit tendons after Prolotherapy treatment confirmed that Prolotherapy stimulates connective tissue repair. This study was published in the journal, *Connective Tissue Research*.[275] Another landmark study was published in 1987 in the prestigious journal *Lancet* by Dr. Thomas Dorman. The study demonstrated the effectiveness of using Prolotherapy to treat back pain.[276] Interestingly, Dr. Dorman was Dr. Neustadt's mentor. Dr. Neustadt spent more than three hundred hours studying directly with Dr. Dorman at Dr. Dorman's private clinic, the Paracelsus Clinic in Kent, Washington (www.paracelsusclinic.com).

More recently, in 2005, the Mayo Clinic featured Prolotherapy in its *Health Letter* publication, which stated that Prolotherapy stimulates tissue growth and is used for tendon and ligament pain.[277] Numerous clinical trials have proven Prolotherapy to be helpful in the treatment of musculoskeletal pain, and Prolotherapy has been endorsed and approved by the American Association of Orthopaedic Medicine and the Florida Academy of Pain Management.

Appendix B

Nutraceuticals Used in Treatment Plans

N-ACETYL-CYSTEINE (NAC) 900 mg, 120 capsules, by Designs for Health. Each capsule contains 1,000 mg NAC.

ACTIVATED CHARCOAL 280 mg 100 cap by MMS Pro. Serving Size: 2 capsules. Servings per Container: 50. Amount per Serving: Charcoal 560 mg. Other Ingredients: Gelatin (capsule). Caution: The high absorbency of Activated Charcoal may reduce the effectiveness of oral medications. Consult with a healthcare professional before taking charcoal capsules with medications. Activated Charcoal is recommended for short-term use only. *Activated Charcoal may cause black stools.* Keep this product out of the reach of children. This package is not child resistant and is not suitable for homes with small children. Double safety sealed with a printed outer shrinkwrap and a printed inner bottle freshness seal. Do not use if either seal is broken or missing. Activated Charcoal contains many small chambers and cavities that "capture" or bind up unwanted materials. The charcoal then carries it safely through the digestive system. MMS Pro uses only the highest quality U.S.P. activated charcoal. Each raw material lot is carefully controlled and tested to ensure safety and purity.

ALPHA LIPOIC ACID by Vital Nutrients, 60 caps. Each capsule contains 300 mg alpha lipoic acid. Take two capsules daily.

AN-30 60 capsules by Nutritional Biochemistry, Inc. Each two capsules contains vitamin C (as ascorbic acid and ascorbyl palmitate) 5 mg, vitamin D (as cholecalciferol) 200 IU, calcium (as calcium citrate) 100 mg, zinc (as zinc picolinate) 28 mg, copper (as copper gluconate) 2 mg.

BCAA POWDER Powder by Pure Encapsulations, 227 grams. Contains 3,000 mg of branched chain amino acids per scoop (L-leucine 1,500 mg; L-isoleucine 750 mg; L-valine 750 mg).

BERBERINE FORTE by Nutritional Biochemistry, Inc. 30 capsules. Many studies have shown plant extracts are equally effective, and in some cases more effective, than prescription antibiotics for their ability to kill bacteria. Additionally, unlike prescription antibiotics, many plant extracts also have antifungal activities. In Traditional Chinese Medicine, *Coptis chinensis* (Coptis) has been used to treat many infectious diseases. Coptis is high in Berberine content. Berberine has been shown to be helpful in bacterial, fungal, and viral infections. Berberine sulfate and Coptis rhizome have demonstrated significant in vitro antimicrobial activity against a wide range of bacterial, fungal, and protozoal micro-organisms, including *Klebsiella*, *Clostridium*, *Pseudomonas*, *Proteus*, *Salmonella*, *Shigella*, *Staphylococcus*, *Streptococcus*, *Vibrio*, *Candida*, *Cryptococcus*, and *Entamoeba* species. Berberine and Coptis inhibit the in vitro growth of a number of *Candida* species. Each capsule contains 100 mg Goldenseal Extract (*Hydrastis canadensis*, 5% hydrastine), 200 mg Goldenthread (*Coptis chinensis*) root extract 4:1, 100 mg Barberry (*Berberis vulgaris*) root extract 4:1, and 5 mg Vitamin C (as Ascorbyl Palmitate) in a vegetarian capsule. Contains no binders or fillers, yeast, wheat, gluten, soy protein, milk/dairy, corn, sodium, sugar, starch, artificial coloring, preservatives, or flavoring.

BIOTIN-8 by Thorne Research. Each capsule contains 8,000 mcg of biotin.

BUFFERED VITAMIN C 1,000 mg, ninety tablets, by Vitaline Formulas. Supplement Facts: serving size one tablet. Servings per container: ninety. Amount per serving: Vitamin C (ascorbic acid) 1 g. Other Ingredients: Stearic acid, calcium carbonate, magnesium stearate, silicon dioxide, hydroxypropyl methylcellulose, and titanium dioxide. Vitaline C.T.R. products are formulated in a special inert porous matrix which allows for a gradual release of active ingredients over a prolonged period of time coinciding with natural biological absorption processes. Notes: If pregnant, nursing, or taking prescription drugs, consult your health care practitioner prior to use. Store in a cool, dry place. Tamper-evident packaging for your protection.

CAL/MAG 90 chew by Rx Vitamins. Ingredients: two chewable tablets contain Calcium (as amino acid chelate) 250 mg, Magnesium (as amino acid chelate) 50 mg. Calories 10, Total Carbohydrate 2 g, Sugars 2 g. Other ingredients: Fructose, Silica, Natural vanilla, Whole food complex—Broccoli, Carrot, Spirulina, Chlorella, Apple, Black Currant. Contains no yeast, dairy, eggs, gluten, corn, soy or wheat, starch, salt, artificial color, or preservatives.

CALCIUM (MCHA), 300 mg, 180 vcaps, by Pure Encapsulations. Each capsule contains Calcium (microcrystalline hydroxyapatite) (bovine) 300 mg.

CARLSON'S COD LIVER OIL by Carlson's Laboratory. One teaspoon delivers Vitamin A 700-1200 IU, Vitamin D 400 IU, Vitamin E (as d-Alpha tocopherol) 10 IU, ALA (alpha-linoleic acid) 40–60 mg, DHA (docosahexaenoic acid) 500–590 mg, EPA (eicosapentaenoic acid) 360–500 mg.

CHEWQ 100 mg, sixty chewtabs, by Crayhon Research. Supplement Facts: serving size, one chewtab. Servings per container, sixty. Amount per serving: Calories 4, Total Carbohydrates 1 g, Coenzyme Q10 (ubidecarenone USP) 100 mg. Other Ingredients: Xylitol, gamma-cyclodextrin, natural orange flavor, magnesium stearate and silicon dioxide. This product does not contain animal products, preservatives, trans fats, or artificial colors. Keep bottle tightly closed. Store in a cool, dry place at a controlled room temperature between 15–30° C (59–86° F). Chew one chewtab with or after a meal.

COFACTOR B, thirty capsules, by Nutritional Biochemistry, Inc. This dietary supplement was formulated by Dr. Neustadt. Each capsule contains vitamin C 7 mg, vitamin B1 (thiamin) 100 mg, vitamin B2 (riboflavin) 100 mg, vitamin B3 (niacin as niacinamide) 100 mg, vitamin B6 (pyridoxine as pyridoxine HCl) 100 mg, folic acid 400 mcg, vitamin B12 (methylcobalamin) 100 mcg, biotin 100 mcg, vitamin B5 (pantothenic acid as calcium pantothenate) 100 mg, choline (as choline bitartrate) 75 mg, inositol 75 mg and PABA (para amino benzoic acid) 30 mg, in a vegetarian capsule. Contains no binders or fillers. Contains *no* yeast, wheat, gluten, soy protein, milk/dairy, corn, sodium, sugar, starch, artificial coloring, preservatives, or flavoring. Note: High doses of B vitamins can change the urine to a bright yellow and alter the smell. This is not toxic and is normal.

CURCUMIN PRO 450 mg 60 tabs by MMS Pro. Curcumin Pro contains a standardized extract of Turmeric (*Curcuma longa*) containing 95% Curcuminoids. This is the highest potency Curcuminoid extract available. Turmeric rhizome has traditionally been used as a digestive aid. Recent research has shown that curcuminoids provide potent antioxidant protection, and as a treatment for irritable bowel disease, and protection against cognitive decline caused by oxidative stress. Each tablet contains 450 mg Turmeric extract standardized to 95% curcuminoids in a base of 50 mg Turmeric root. Take one tablet twice daily.

CUSTOMIZED AMINO ACID BLEND from Metabolic Maintenance. This is a specially-formulated blend of amino acids based on your lab results that is intended to correct amino acid imbalances. Results may vary, but most patients report positive response in 3–14 days.

DIM ENHANCED DELIVERY SYSTEM 120 caps. DIM Enhanced Delivery System contains BioResponse DIM, a unique formulation containing pure Diindilymethane, an indole. Indoles are plant compounds with health promoting properties, found in cruciferous vegetables such as broccoli, cabbage, cauliflower and brussel sprouts. DIM has been shown to help regulate and promote a more efficient metabolism of estrogen, and an optimal ratio of estrogen metabolites. Four Capsules Provide: BioResponse DIM 300 mg (A patented diindolylmethane complex: starch, DIM (25% min.), Vitamin E succcinate, phosphatidylcholine, silica). Other ingredients: Cellulose, carbowax, silicon dioxide. Note: Harmless changes in urine color may occur.

EGCG 250 mg 60 tabs, by Designs for Health. Each capsule contains Green Tea (decaffeinated) 500 mg (Camellia sinensis) (leaves) (standardized to contain 50% epigallocatechin gallate). Other Ingredients: Rice flour, magnesium stearate, microcrystalline cellulose. Store in a cool, dry place. Keep out of reach of children. This product does not contain wheat, yeast, soy protein, gluten, eggs, dairy, corn, artificial colors, flavors, sugars, or preservatives.

ENTEROPRO 60 capsules by Longevity Science. EnteroPro is a powerful combination of six beneficial probiotic organisms, with a total of ten billion total organisms per capsule at time of manufacture. The special enteric coating of the capsule assures maximum potency by delivering the organisms directly to the intestines, avoiding the loss of potency caused by contact with stomach acid. Each capsule contains L. acidophilus DDS-1 1.67 billion, B. bifidum 1.67 billion, L. bulgaricus 1.67 billion, L. casei 1.67 billion, L. planatarum 1.67

billion, L. salivarius 1.67 billion, Frutafit Inulin 50 mg. L. salivarius, L. plantarum, and L. casei are especially effective at reducing urnary indican concentrations.

EVENING PRIMROSE OIL 500 mg 120 gels. Each softgel contains Evening Primrose oil 500 mg, including Omega 6 FA 400-410 mg Gamma linolenic (GLA) 45-50 mg, Linoleic acid 340-360 mg. Free of all common plant and animal allergens, no hydrogenated oils, preservatives or other additives.

EXTREME SPORTS DRINK by Nutritional Biochemistry, Inc. Amount per Serving % Daily Values*, Calories 25, Calories from fat 0, Total fat 0 g 0%, Cholesterol 0 mg 0%, Sodium 70 mg 3%, Total Carbohydrate 5 g 2%, Dietary Fiber 0 g 0%, Sugars 5 g, Protein 0 g, Vitamin C 1,000 mg 1667%, (as Ascorbic Acid and Sodium Ascorbate), Thiamine 15 mg 1,000% (as Thiamine Mononitrate), Riboflavin 10 mg 588%, Niacin (as Niacinamide) 30 mg 150%, Vitamin B-6 (as Pyridoxine HCl) 25 mg 1250%, Folate (as Folic Acid) 15 mcg 4%, Vitamin B-12 15 mcg 250%, (as Methylcobalamin), Biotin 50 mcg 17%, Pantothenic Acid 75 mg 750% (as d-Calcium Pantothenate), Other ingredients: fructose, glycine, natural flavors. Amount per Serving % Daily Values*: Calcium (as Calcium Citrate) 75 mg 8%, Phosphorus 40 mg 4% (as Potassium Phosphate), Magnesium 100 mg 25% (as Magnesium Glycinate), Zinc (as Zinc Citrate) 1 mg 7%, Copper (as Copper Citrate) 0.1 mg 5%, Manganese 2 mg 100% (as Manganese Glycinate), Chromium 75 mcg 63% (as Chromium Picolinate), Potassium 99 mg 3% (as Potassium Phosphate) L-Carnitine 2000 mg ** (as L-Carnitine tartrate), Acetyl L-Carnitine 2000 mg ** (as Acetyl L-Carnitine HCl), Alpha Ketoglutaric Acid 25 mg **, Stevia leaf extract 60 mg ** (*Stevia rebaudiana*, standardized to 90% steviosides), * Percent Daily Values are based on a 2,000 calorie diet. ** Daily value not established.

FENUCHROME ninety capsules, by Nutritional Biochemistry, Inc. Each three capsules contains vitamin C (as ascorbic acid and ascorbyl palmitate) 240 mg, magnesium (as magnesium amino acid blend), chromium (as chromium picolinate) 100 mcg, Cinnulin PF (*Cinnamomum cassia* bark, water extract, 20:1, standardized to 1% trimeric and tetrameric type-A polymers) 500 mg, Fenugreek seed extract (*Trigonella foenum-graecum*, 25:1) 600 mg.

FERROSOLVE 30 capsules by Nutritional Biochemistry, Inc. Each capsule contains 45 mg iron (as Ferrochel™ amino acid chelate) and 70 mg glycine. The form of iron in this formula is highly absorbable, with approximately 75% of it being absorbed. Other ingredients: vegetarian cellulose capsules, magnesium stearate. Contains no yeast, wheat, gluten, sodium, sugar, starch, artificial coloring, preservatives or flavoring. WARNING: Accidental overdose or iron-containing products is a leading cause of fatal poisoning in children under six. Keep this product out of reach of children. In case of accidental overdose, call a poison control center immediately.

FRUITS N GREENS 180 gm, by NewMark. Supplemental facts: Serving size one tablespoon (6 g). Servings per container, thirty. Amount per serving: Calories 20, Total fat 0 g, Saturated fat 0 g, Trans fat 0 g, Cholesterol 0 mg, Sodium 45 mg, Total carbohydrate 4 g, Dietary fiber 2 g, Sugars 1 g, Protein 1 g, Vitamin A (100% as beta-carotene) 500 IU, Vitamin C 2 mg, Calcium 40 mg, Iron 1 mg, Vitamin D 130 IU, Vitamin K 55 mcg, Riboflavin (B2) .07 mg, Vitamin B6 .06 mg, Iodine 7 mcg, Magnesium 16 mg, Manganese .9 mg, Chromium 5 mcg, Molybdenum 6 mcg, Ingredients: Organic spinach, Organic blueberry, Organic kale, Organic parsley, Organic cranberry, Organic red cabbage*, Organic green cabbage*, Organic broccoli*, Organic brussel sprouts*, Organic okra*, Organic papaya*, Organic rose hips*, Organic pomegranate*, Organic Concord grapes*, Organic oats*, Organic brown rice*, Organic turmeric*, Organic ginger*, Organic cinnamon*, Organic chicory*. Probiotic blend for *L. casei, L. plantarum, L. salivarius, L. acidophilus, L. rhamnosus, S. thermophilus, B. bifidum, B. infantis, B. longum, B. breve.* *Ingredients cultured with the ten listed probiotic species, one billion per serving at the time of manufacture. Warning: For best results *refrigerate after opening.*

GLUTAMINE RX 200 grams, by Nutritional Biochemistry, Inc. Each teaspoon (one serving) contains 3,000 mg L-glutamine. Contains no binders, fillers, soy, wheat, yeast, preservatives, dairy, starch, artificial coloring, preservatives, or flavoring. 67 Servings per container.

GLYCINE POWDER, by Vital Nutrients, 250 grams. Glycine is an inhibitory neurotransmitter than can help with anxiety. Each half teaspoon contains 2,000 mg glycine.

HOMOCYSTEINE FACTORS by Pure Encapsulations. Each capsule contains vitamins B6, B12, folic acid, and trimethylglycine to decrease your homocysteine, which is an independent risk factor for cardiovascular disease, dementia, osteoporosis, and other chronic degenerative conditions. *Refrigerate after opening.* Take one capsule twice daily with food.

I-FLORA 4 KIDS 36 gms by Sedona Labs. Supplement Facts: Serving Size 1/4 tsp (625 mg). Servings per container 57, containing Proprietary blend 49 mg Lactobacillus acidophilis, Lactobacillus rhamnosus, Bifidobacterium infantis, Lactobacillus paracasei, Bifidobacterium bifidum, Bifidobacterium longum. Other ingredients: Rice starch. Each serving of I-Flora 4 Kids contains four billion viable cells of the most researched probiotic strains used for children.

IMMUNOPRO 300 grams. Each scoop (5 grams) contains: Calories 20, Total Fat 0.3 g, Cholesterol 5 mg, Sodium 10 mg, Potassium 30 mg, Total Carbohydrate 0.3 g, Dietary Fiber 0 g, Sugars 0 g, Protein 4 g, Calcium 20 mg, Immunoglobulins 645 mg, Lactoferrin 170 mg. The immunoglobulins and lactoferrin are immune boosting. A sweetener may be added for flavor. Keep container closed. Store in a cool, dry place. Serving scoop enclosed in jar.

K+2 POTASSIUM 300 mg, 120 caps, by Designs for Health. Each capsule contains potassium 300 mg as potassium glycinate complex, potassium bicarbonate. Other ingredients: Gelatin, stearic acid, magnesium stearate. Take one capsule daily with food.

L-HISTIDINE 600 mg 50 caps, by Pure Encapsulations. Caution: Those with elevated Histidine or histamine levels should not take L-Histidine supplementation. These may include manic-depressives, those with schizophrenia or problems with chronic allergies, pregnant women, or women with PMS. Individuals who have hypertension should exercise caution, and those with peptic ulcers and excessive gastric juices should avoid Histidine supplementation.

LIQUID PEDIATRIC 6 OZ by NF Formulas. One teaspoon provides: Vitamin A (palmitate) 1667 i.u., Vitamin C (ascorbic acid) 50mg, Vitamin B-1 .8 mg, Vitamin B-2 .8 mg, Vitamin B-3 3.3 mg, Iron (ferric ammonium citrate) 3.3 mg, Vitamin D-3 167 i.u., Vitamin E 10 i.u., Vitamin B-6 1 mg, Folic acid 67 mcg, Vitamin B-12 1.67 mcg, Iodine 25 mcg, Magnesium (chloride) 4.2 mg, Zinc sulfate 3.3 mg, Copper sulfate .3 mg, Biotin 67 mcg, Vitamin B-5 1.67 mg, Chlorine (chloride) 10 mg, Inositol 7 mg, Potassium (citrate) 8.3 mg, Manganese (sulfate) .8 mg, Vitamin B-10 (PABA) .3 mg, Molybdenum (trioxide) 83 mcg, Vandadium (peroxtoxide) 83 mcg, Chromium (chloride) 33 mcg, Selenium (sodium selenite) 33 mcg. Shake well before each use.

LIVER SUPPORT 120 caps, by Vital Nutrients. Liver Support contains per two capsules: Dandelion Root Extract 4:1 200mg, Artichoke Leaf Extract 6:1 200mg, Curcumin Extract 20:1 200mg, Milk Thistle Seed Extract 200mg, (Silybin, Silicristin, Silidianin, Silymarin min. 80% by HPLC), Schisandra Extract 20:1 100mg, Bupleurum Extract 10:1 100mg, Rehmannia Extract 6:1 100mg, Choline Bitartrate 160mg, Methionine (L Form) 100mg. Other ingredients: Gelatin capsule, calcium carbonate. May contain Ascorbyl Palmitate and\or Silica. Take two capsules twice daily. *Take one bottle and then discontinue.*

L-METHIONINE 500 mg, one hundred capsules, by Metabolic Maintenance. Each capsule contains Vitamin C (as Ascorbyl Palmitate) 5 mg, L-Methionine 500 mg. Take one capsule daily. (This will be special-ordered for you).

L-TRYPTOPHAN 500mg 120c by Lidtke Technologies. Each capsule contains L-Tryptophan, USP 500mg. Other ingredients: Gelatin capsule, vegetable stearic acid, plant cellulose, silica.

MAG-10, thirty capsules, by Nutritional Biochemistry, Inc. Each capsule contains 250 mg magnesium (as magnesium amino acid chelate) and 100 mg coenzyme Q10 (CoQ10) in a vegetarian capsule. Contains no binders or fillers. Contains *no* yeast, wheat, gluten, soy protein, milk/dairy, corn, sodium, sugar, starch, artificial coloring, preservatives, or flavoring.

MITOFORTE 120 capsules, by Nutritional Biochemistry, Inc. Each four capsules contains 800 mg L-carnitine, 800 mg Acetyl-L-Carnitine, 600 mg Alpha-lipoic Acid, 200 mcg biotin, 200 mg N-acetylcysteine, 200 mg Turmeric (*Curcuma longa*) root standardized to 95% curcuminoids in a vegetarian capsule. Contains no binders or fillers. Contains *no* yeast, wheat, gluten, soy protein, milk/dairy, corn, sodium, sugar, starch, artificial coloring, preservatives, or flavoring. This formula was created by Dr. Neustadt after his extensive research into the basic biochemistry of health and disease. It helps increase energy, improve mental acuity and alertness, and decrease blood sugar and triglycerides, as well as providing powerful antioxidant protection to the cells.

NATTOPINE by Nutritional Biochemistry, Inc., sixty capsules. Each two capsules contains soy-derived nattokinase 3650 fibrinolytic units (FU), pine bark extract (*Pinus massoniana* standardized to 95% proanthocyanidins) 300 mg, vitamin C as ascorbyl palmitate 10 mg. Nattokinase decreases tendency to form blood clots by decreasing fibrinogen, decreases blood viscosity ("thins the blood"), and can decrease blood pressure. Pine bark extract contains powerful antioxidants (proanthocyanidins) to help prevent and reverse free radical damage.

NIASAFE by Thorne Research. Niasafe contains the safer, non-flushing form of niacin— inositol hexaniacinate. Niacin reduces VLDL, LDL, Lp(a), triglycerides, and fibrinogen. It also increases HDL.

OSTEO-K 180 capsules, by Nutritional Biochemistry, Inc. The nutrients in this formula have been shown in multiple clinical trials to increase bone mineral density up to about 10% and decrease fracture risk up to 81%. Each six capsules contains Vitamin D 2,000 IU (as D-3, Cholecalciferol), Vitamin K 45,000 mcg (as K-2, menaquinone-4), Calcium 1,200 mg (as Calcium Citrate/Malate), magnesium (as amino acid chelate) 300 mg and boron 1 mg. Other ingredients: vegetarian cellulose capsules. This product contains NO yeast, wheat, gluten, soy protein, milk/dairy, corn, sodium, sugar, starch, artificial coloring, preservatives or flavoring. This product is hypoallergenic. <u>CAUTION: Do not take this product if you are on anticoagulant medicine (e.g., warfarin)</u>.

PARA-GARD 120 caps, by Integrative Therapeutics, Inc. Each three capsules contain Berberine Sulfate 300 mg, Grapefruit (Citrus x paradisi) Seed Extract 300 mg, Gentian (Gentiana lutea) Root 225 mg, 4:1 Extract, Goldenseal (Hydrastis canadensis) Root 150 mg Extract 5% Total Alkaloids, Black Walnut (Juglans nigra) Green Outer Hull 150 mg 4:1 Extract, Garlic (Allium sativum) Bulb 150 mg, Extract 0.8% Allicin, Jamaica Quassia (Picrasma excelsa) Bark 150 mg 4:1 Extract, Sweet Wormwood (Artemisia annua) 150 mg Aerial Parts/ Other Ingredients: Natural polysaccharide capsule, magnesium stearate, microcrystalline cellulose, and silicon dioxide. Contains no: milk, yeast, gluten, corn, soy, or ingredients of animal origin. Notes: If taking prescription drugs, consult your health care practitioner prior to use. Keep this product out of reach of children. Store in a cool, dry place. Tamper-evident packaging for your protection. As with any product, discontinue use if adverse effects occur.

PERFUSIA SR by Thorne Research, 180 capsules. Perfusia-SR is a sustained-release formulation of the amino acid L-arginine. Supplementation with L-arginine improves the production of nitric oxide by vascular endothelial cells, which increases vasodilation while inhibiting platelet and monocyte adhesiveness, resulting, for example, in enhanced cardiovascular health. This unique, sustained-release product provides for improved long-term blood levels with twice daily dosing. Each capsule contains 350 mg L-Arginine.

PROMINERALS 90 capsules by Nutritional Biochemistry, Inc. Each 3 capsules contain: Calcium (as Calcium Citrate/malate) 100 mg, Iodine (as Potassium Iodide) 40 mcg, Magnesium (as Magnesium Amino Acid Chelete) 90 mg, Zinc (as Zinc Citrate) 7 mg, Selenium (as L-Selenomethionine) 50 mcg, Copper (as Copper Citrate), 1.3 mg, Manganese (as Manganese Citrate) 5 mg, Chromium (as Chromium Polynicotinate) 66.7 mcg, Molybdenum (as Molybdenum AA Chelate) 30 mcg, Potassium (as Potassium Citrate) 30 mg, Boron (as Boron Citrate) 1 mg, Vanadium (as Vandyl Sulfate) 100 mcg, Vitamin C (as Ascorbyl Palmitate) 6.7 mg. Other ingredients: vegetarian cellulose capsule.

PROTECT DM 30 capsules by Nutritional Biochemistry, Inc. Each capsule contains vitamin C (as ascorbic acid and ascorbyl palmitate) 60 mg, Pine Bark extract (*Pinus massoniana*, standardized to 95% proanthocyanidins) 150 mg, and Turmeric root extract (*Curcuma longa,* standardized to 95% curcuminoids) 250 mg. A recent clinical trial showed significant improvements in blood flow compared to the control group after four weeks of treatment.

PURE L-ASPARTIC ACID 500 mg 100 caps by Montiff. Each capsule contains L-Aspartic Acid 500 mg. Other ingredients: Microcrystalline Cellulose, Magnesim Stearate, Silicon Dioxide, Gelatin. Contains no Starch, Corn, Milk, Wheat, Yeast, Sugar, Eggs, Salt, Artificial Colors, Binders, Flavors, Preservatives or fish derivatives.

PURE L-GLUTAMIC ACID 500 mg 100 caps by Montiff. Each capsule contains L-Glutamic Acid 500 mg. Other ingredients: Microcrystalline Cellulose, Magnesium Stearate, Gelatin. Contains no Starch, Corn, Milk, Wheat, Yeast, Sugar, Eggs, Salt, Artificial Colors, Binders, Flavors, Preservatives or fish derivatives.

PURE ORNITHINE-KETOGLUTARATE 500 mg, one hundred capsules, by Montiff. Each capsule contains Ornithine-a-Ketoglutarate 500 mg. Take two capsules per day on with water or fruit juice. Do not take with dairy products.

REJUVAMAG 60 capsules by Nutritional Biochemistry, Inc. Each capsule contains 250 mg magnesium as magnesium amino acid chelate, and 10 mg vitamin C as ascorbyl palmitate.

RESCULPT by Nutritional Biochemistry Incorporated 698 grams. This dietary supplement was formulated by Dr. Neustadt. Each two scoops contain: Calories 85, Calories from fat 0, Total fat 0 g, Cholesterol 0 mg, Sodium 35 mg, Total Carbohydrate 1 g, Dietary Fiber 0 g, Sugars 1 g, Protein 20 g, Vitamin B-6 30 mg (as 50 mg of Pyridoxal-5-Phosphate), Calcium (from whey protein) 95 mg, Phosphorus (from whey protein) 50 mg, Potassium (from whey protein) 100 mg, Stevia leaf extract 50 mg, (Stevia rebaudiana, standardized to 90% steviosides), L-Glutamine 100 mg, L-Alanine 1000 mg, L-Arginine 384 mg, L-Aspartic Acid 2198 mg, L-Cystine 458 mg, L-Glutamic Acid 3511 mg, Glycine 329 mg, L-Histidine 342 mg, L-Isoleucine 1471 mg, L-Leucine 2198 mg, L-Lysine 1895 mg, L-Methionine 404 mg, L-Phenylalanine 595 mg, L-Proline 1300 mg, L-Serine 904 mg, L-Threonine 1427 mg, L-Tryptophan 331 mg, L-Tyrosine 567 mg. L-Valine 1315 mg, This product contains NO yeast, wheat, gluten, added sugar, starch, artificial coloring, preservatives, or flavoring. 98% lactose free. Not expected to cause problems for people with lactose intolerance. Other ingredients: whey protein isolate, natural flavors, lecithin. Contains milk and soy. Note: L-Tryptophan is naturally occurring, not added.

RESVERATROL 200 mg, 120 vcaps, by Pure Encapsulations. Resveratrol is a compound often associated with the health benefits of red wine, because of its powerful antioxidant and cardioprotectant properties. It promotes cardiovascular health through its antioxidant action and its ability to modulate platelet aggregation and arachidonic acid metabolism. Pure Encapsulations Resveratrol is derived from one of the richest known sources, Polygonum cuspidatum, an herb utilized as a nutritional agent for centuries. Resveratrol is standardized to contain 20% total resveratrols and 10% emodin, providing high-potency cardiovascular and antioxidant support. Each VCapsule Contains resveratrol (Polygonum cuspidatum) extract (standardized to contain 20% total resveratrols and 10% emodin) 200 mg. Take two capsules twice daily.

SAMe, 200 mg, thirty tablets, by Designs for Health. Size: thirty tablets—blister pack. Each tablet contains Vitamin B6 (as Pyridoxine HCI) 2 mg, Folic Acid 200 mcg, Vitamin B12 (as Cyanocobalamin) 50 mcg, S-Adenosyl L-Methionine (SAMe) 200 mg. SAMe is important in providing methyl donors for liver detoxification pathways, for proper brain function, and for cardiovascular health.

SUBLINGUAL B-6 4 oz by Designs for Health. Serving Size: one teaspoon (5 ml) Servings Per Container: 23.6. Amount Per Serving: Calories 14, Vitamin B6 50 mg, (as pyridoxine HCl and pyridoxal-5-phosphate), Magnesium 30 mg (as di-magnesium malate), Zinc 5 mg, (as zinc amino acid chelate). Other Ingredients: Vegetable glycerin, deionized water, citric acid, raspberry natural flavor. This product does not contain any milk or dairy, egg, fish, shellfish, tree nuts, peanuts, wheat, gluten, or soy.

SUPER D3, by Allergy Research Group, sixty capsules. Each capsule contains 2,000 IU vitamin D3, 20 IU vitamin E, and 2 mg vitamin C.

SUPER LIQUID FOLATE 1 oz by Designs for Health. Size: 1 ounce/480 drops per bottle. Suggested dose: one or more drops per day. Each drop contains: Folic acid (proprietary delivery system) 800 mcg, B12 (hydroxycobalamin) 6 mcg. Other ingredients: distilled water, buffered potassium sorbate. Super Liquid Folate contains a highly absorbable form of folic acid that assures maximal absorption and assimilation. Our proprietary formula is three times better absorbed than other liquid suspensions of folic acid. This is due to our unique manufacturing process, which makes folic acid completely soluble in water.

SUPREME FEM MULTIVITAMIN (WITH IRON) 120 capsules, by Nutritional Biochemistry, Inc. Servings per bottle: 30. Each 4 capsules contain Vitamin A 10000 IU (as Beta Carotene from Betatene® Mixed Carotenoids), Vitamin C 1000 mg (as Ascorbic Acid and Ascorbyl Palmitate), Vitamin D-3 (as Cholecalciferol) 1000 IU,. Vitamin E 400 IU (as d-Alpha Tocopheryl Succinate), Vitamin K 120 mcg, Thiamin (as Thiamin Mononitrate) 50 mg. Riboflavin 50 mg, Niacin (as Niacinamide) 75 mg. Vitamin B-6 (as Pyridoxine HCl) 50 mg, Folate (as Folic Acid) 400 mcg, Vitamin B-12 (as Methylcobalamin) 450 mcg, Biotin 400 mcg, Pantothenic Acid 100 mg (as Calcium Pantothenate), Calcium 200 mg (from Calcium Citrate/Malate), Iron 8 mg (as Ferrochel® amino acid chelate), Iodine (from Atlantic Kelp) 100 mcg, Magnesium 200 mg (from Magnesium Amino Acid Chelate), Zinc (from Zinc Amino Acid Chelate) 15 mg, Selenium 200 mcg (from L-Selenomethionine), Copper 1.5 mg (from Copper Amino Acid Chelate), Manganese 5 mg (from Manganese Amino Acid Chelate), Chromium 200 mcg (from Chromium Picolinate), Molybdenum 50 mcg (from Molybdenum Amino Acid Chelate), Potassium 99 mg (from Potassium Citrate), Vanadium 200 mcg (from Vanadyl Sulfate), Boron (from Boron Citrate) 1 mg, Alpha Carotene 190 mcg (from Betatene® Mixed Carotenoids), Zeaxanthin 38 mcg (from Betatene® Mixed Carotenoids), Cryptoxanthin 45 mcg (from Betatene® Mixed Carotenoids), Choline 50 mg (as Choline Bitartrate), Citrus Bioflavonoid Complex 200 mg, CoEnzyme Q10 10 mg, Grape seed extract 10 mg (*Vitis vinifera* standardized to 95% proanthocyanins), Turmeric root extract 40 mg (*Curcuma longa* standardized to 95% curcuminoids). Other ingredients: vegetarian cellulose capsules.

SUPREME MULTIVITAMIN (WITHOUT IRON), 120 capsules. Servings per bottle: thirty. Each four capsules contains Vitamin A 10,000 IU (as Beta Carotene from Betatene Mixed Carotenoids), Vitamin C 1,000 mg (as Ascorbic Acid and Ascorbyl Palmitate), Vitamin D-3 (as Cholecalciferol) 1,000 IU, Vitamin E 400 IU (as d-Alpha Tocopheryl Succinate), Vitamin K 120 mcg, Thiamin (as Thiamin Mononitrate) 50 mg. Riboflavin 50 mg, Niacin (as Niacinamide) 75 mg. Vitamin B-6 (as Pyridoxine HCl) 50 mg, Folate (as Folic Acid) 400 mcg, Vitamin B-12 (as Methylcobalamin) 450 mcg, Biotin 400 mcg, Pantothenic Acid 100 mg (as Calcium Pantothenate), Calcium 200 mg (from Calcium Citrate/Malate), Iodine (from Atlantic Kelp) 100 mcg, Magnesium 200 mg (from Magnesium Amino Acid Chelate), Zinc (from Zinc Amino Acid Chelate) 15 mg, Selenium 200 mcg (from L-Selenomethionine), Copper 1.5 mg (from Copper Amino Acid Chelate), Manganese 5 mg (from Manganese Amino Acid Chelate), Chromium 200 mcg (from Chromium Picolinate), Molybdenum 50 mcg (from Molybdenum Amino Acid Chelate), Potassium 99 mg (from Potassium Citrate), Vanadium 200 mcg (from Vanadyl Sulfate), Boron (from Boron Citrate) 1 mg, Alpha Carotene 190 mcg (from Betatene Mixed Carotenoids), Zeaxanthin 38 mcg (from Betatene Mixed Carotenoids), Cryptoxanthin 45 mcg (from Betatene Mixed Carotenoids), Choline 50 mg (as Choline Bitartrate), Citrus Bioflavonoid Complex 200 mg, CoEnzyme Q10 10 mg, Grape seed extract 10 mg (*Vitis vinifera* standardized to 95% proanthocyanins), Turmeric root extract 40 mg (*Curcuma longa* standardized to 95% curcuminoids). Other ingredients: vegetarian cellulose capsules.

TAURINE POWDER, 1,500 mg, 100 grams, by Designs for Health. Each quarter teaspoon contains 1,500 mg taurine.

TYROSINE 1g, sixty tablets, by Designs for Health. Each tablet contains Vitamin C (as ascorbic acid) 50 mg, and Tyrosine 1,000 mg. Other Ingredients: Microcrystalline cellulose, croscarmellose sodium, magnesium stearate, stearic acid. Store in a cool, dry place. Keep out of reach of children. This product does not contain wheat, yeast, soy protein, gluten, eggs, dairy, corn, artificial colors, flavors, sugars, or preservatives.

ULTRA PROTEIN PLUS - CHOCOLATE ALMOND POWDER 948 gms. Serving size: 1 heaping scoop, 31.6 grams. Servings per container: approximately 30. Each serving contains: Calories 92, Total carbohydrates 7.6 g, Sugars (as Fructose) 5 g, Soluble Fiber 1 g, Protein 18 g. Each serving provides approximately: Vitamin A Palmitate/Beta-Carotene 6,105 IU, Vitamin C (Abscorbic Acid, Corn Free) 260 mg, Vitamin D-3 25 IU, Vitamin E (as d-alpha tocopheryl) 100 IU, Vitamin B-1 (Thiamin HCl) 24 mg, Vitamin B-2 (Riboflavin) 12 mg, Niacin/Niacinamide 43 mg, Pantothenic Acid (d-Calcium Pantothenate) 125 mg, Vitamin B-6 24 mg (Pyridoxine HCI/Pyridoxal-5-Phosphate Complex), Folic Acid 200 mcg, Vitamin B-12 (on Ion Exchange Resin) 25 mcg, Biotin 75 mcg, Pantothenic Acid (d-Calcium Pantothenate) 125 mg, Calcium (Citrate/Ascorbate Complex) 112 mg, Iodine (Kelp) 45 mcg, Magnesium (Aspartate/Ascorbate Complex) 115 mg, Zinc (Amino Acid Chelate) 5 mg, Selenium (Organic Selenium in Krebs* Cycle and Kelp) 45 mcg, Manganese (Aspartate Complex) 4.5 mg, Chromium GTF 45 mcg (Organically bound with GTF activity - low allergenicity), Molybdenum (Krebs*) 23 mcg, Potassium (Aspartate Complex) 22 mg, Choline citrate/Bitartrate 34 mg, Inositol 23 mg, Citrus Bioflavonoid Complex 23 mg, PABA (Para-Aminobenzoic Acid) 11 mg, Vanadium (Krebs*) 11 mcg, Boron (Aspartate/Citrate Complex) 0.3 mg, Trace Elements (from Sea Vegetation) approx 20 mcg, L-Cysteine/N-Acetyl-L-Cysteine 45 mg, Betaine HCl 34 mg. Typical Amino Acid Profile: Glutamic Acid 3565 mg, Aspartic Acid 2215 mg, Arginine 1620 mg, Lysine 1480 mg, Leucine 1440 mg, Phenylalanine 990 mg, Serine 970 mg, Valine 940 mg, Alanine 850 mg, Glycine 830 mg, Isoleucine 830 mg, Proline 810 mg, Threonine 740 mg, Tyrosine 740 mg, Histidine 500 mg, Cysteine 220 mg, Methionine 200 mg, Tryptophan 180 mg. Other Ingredients: Yellow pea protein, Fructose, Dutch cocoa, BeFlora soluble fiber, Natural almond flavor.

URI FORMULA. Each alcohol-free capsule contains concentrated extracts of Garlic bulb (*Allium sativum*) 40mg, Osha root (*Ligusticum porterii*) 34 mg, Lomatium root (*Lomatium dissectum*) 30 mg, Grindelia floral bud (*Grindelia robusta*) 22 mg, Irish Moss (*Chondrus crispus*) 20 mg, Hyssop flowers (*Hyssopus officinalis*) 10 mg, Barberry root (*Berberis vulgaris*) 8 mg, Oregon Grape root (*Barberis aquifolium*) 8 mg, Goldenseal rhizome (*Hydrastis canadensis*) 8 mg, Mullen leaf (*Verbascum olympicum*) 8 mg, Lobelia herb and seed (*Lobelia inflata*) 6 mg, St. John's Wort (*Hypericum perforatum*) flower bud 6 mg, *Echinacea purpurea* root 4 mg, *Echinacea purpurea* flowering top 4 mg, *Echinacea angustifolia* root 3 mg, *Echinacea purpurea* seed 0.7 mg.

VITAL MIXED ASCORBATES by Pharmax, 250 grams. Each scoop (5 grams) contains, Vitamin C 2,000mg (as freeze-dried mineral: ascorbic acid 3:1), Magnesium 40mg, (as freeze-dried magnesium ascorbate), Calcium (as calcium ascorbate) 40mg, Potassium 180mg, (as freeze-dried potassium ascorbate: potassium bicarbonate 3:1), Manganese 10mg, (as freeze-dried manganese ascorbate), Zinc (as freeze-dried zinc ascorbate) 7.7mg, Apricot concentrate 10:1 290mg, (*Prunus armeniaca*), Blackcurrant concentrate 10:1, 290mg, (*Ribes nigrum*), Blueberry concentrate 10:1, 290mg (*Vaccinium myrtillus*), Blackcherry concentrate 10:1, 100mg (*Prunus cerasus*). Vitamin C and the flavonoids in the various plant extracts in this formula decrease inflammation and oxidative stress.

VITAMIN C POWDER by Pharmax, 250 grams. Each scoop contains, Vitamin C 940 mg, (as freeze-dried magnesium ascorbate), Magnesium 60mg, (as freeze-dried magnesium ascorbate).

VITAMIN D3 5000 IU 60 vcaps by Pure Encapsulations. A hypo-allergenic dietary supplement. Each capsule contains Vitamin D3 5,000 IU. Other Ingredients: hypo-allergenic plant fiber, vegetable capsule. Store sealed in a cool dry area. Keep out of the reach of children. Tamper resistant: Use only if safety seal is intact. This encapsulated product contains no hidden coatings, excipients, binders, fillers, shellacs, artificial colors or fragrance. Contains no dairy, wheat, yeast, gluten, corn, sugar, starch, soy, preservatives or hydrogenated oils. Supports bone, cardiovascular, colon and cellular health.

VITAMIN E MIXED TOCOPH 400 IU 100 count by Vital Nutrients. Natural Vitamin E with D-Alpha and Mixed Tocopherols. Each softgel contains: Vitamin E 400 400 i.u., d-alpha tocopherol 268.456 mg, d-Beta, d-Gamma and d-Delta tocopherols 60 mg. Other ingredients: Soybean oil, gelatin. Contains no coatings, binders, fillers, or dairy, wheat, eggs, yeast, commercial sugars, starch, preservatives, or hydrogenated oil.

About the Authors

John Neustadt, ND received his naturopathic medical degree from Bastyr University. Dr. Neustadt also earned degrees in Literature (cum laude) from the University of California, San Diego, and Botany (departmental honors) from the University of Washington. He worked as a journalist in Chile and San Francisco before returning to naturopathic medical school. Dr. Neustadt is medical director of Montana Integrative Medicine (MIM) and president and CEO of Nutritional Biochemistry, Incorporated (NBI) and NBI Testing and Consulting Corp (NBITC), in Bozeman, Mont. In 2008, Dr. Neustadt was voted Best Doctor amongst all physicians in the Best of Bozeman survey. This was the first time a naturopathic doctor had ever won this distinction. Dr. Neustadt is coauthor with Steve Pieczenik, MD, PhD of the books, *A Revolution in Health through Nutritional Biochemistry* and *A Revolution in Health Part 2: How to Take Charge of Your Health*. He also wrote the book, *Thriving through Dialysis*, with Jonathan Wright, MD. Dr. Neustadt is an editor of the textbook *Laboratory Evaluations for Integrative and Functional Medicine* and a frequent contributor to the journal *Integrative Medicine: A Clinician's Journal*. He is on the editorial advisory board of the *Journal of Prolotherapy* and *Remedies* magazine. Dr. Neustadt has published more than one hundred research reviews and is a frequent guest on national and local radio health programs.

Steve Pieczenik, MD, PhD trained in psychiatry at Harvard and has an MD from Cornell University Medical College and a PhD in International Relations from Massachusetts Institute of Technology. He twice won the prestigious Harry C. Solomon Award for outstanding research in psychiatry at Harvard Medical College, received a National Institute of Mental Health (NIMH) five-year fellowship award, and was Director of International Activities at the NIMH. He is a board-certified psychiatrist and was a board examiner in psychiatry and neurology. Dr. Pieczenik was Deputy Assistant Secretary of State under Presidents Nixon, Ford, Carter, Reagan and Bush Sr. He was a Senior Consultant to the RAND Corporation and the U.S. Department of Defense, and is an internationally recognized crisis manager and hostage negotiator. He is chairman of the board of NBI and NBITC. Dr. Pieczenik co-created twenty-six New York Times bestselling books, including *Tom Clancy's Op-Center* and *Tom Clancy's NetForce*.

Contact Information

Readers may contact Montana Integrative Medicine, Nutritional Biochemistry, Inc (NBI) and NBI Testing and Consulting Corporation (NBITC) to inquire about testing and treatment options, as well as collaborative business and educational opportunities.

Montana Integrative Medicine

1087 Stoneridge Drive, Suite 1
Bozeman, MT 59718
Phone: 406-582-0034
www.montanaim.com
info@montanaim.com

Nutritional Biochemistry, Inc (NBI) and NBI Testing and Consulting Corporation (NBITC)

1087 Stoneridge Drive, Suite 1
Bozeman, MT 59718
Toll free: 800-624-1416
www.nbihealth.com | www.nbitesting.com
info@ nbihealth.com | info@nbitesting.com

References

1.   Garrod AE. The incidence of alkaptonuria: a study in chemical individuality. *Lancet.* 1902;11:1616-1620.

2.   Williams R. *Biochemical Individuality: the basis for the genotrophic concept.* New York: McGraw-Hill; 1998.

3.   Ames BN, Elson-Schwab I, Silver EA. High-dose vitamin therapy stimulates variant enzymes with decreased coenzyme binding affinity (increased K(m)): relevance to genetic disease and polymorphisms. *Am J Clin Nutr.* Apr 2002;75(4):616-658.

4.   Ames BN. The metabolic tune-up: metabolic harmony and disease prevention. *J Nutr.* May 2003;133(5 Suppl 1):1544S-1548S.

5.   Ames BN, Liu J. Delaying the Mitochondrial Decay of Aging with Acetylcarnitine. Vol 1033; 2004:108-116.

6.   Ames BN, Shigenaga MK, Hagen TM. Oxidants, antioxidants, and the degenerative diseases of aging. *Proc Natl Acad Sci U S A.* Sep 1 1993;90(17):7915-7922.

7.   Xu F, Ding H. A new kinetic model for heterogeneous (or spatially confined) enzymatic catalysis: Contributions from the fractal and jamming (overcrowding) effects. *Applied Catalysis A: General.* 2007;317(1):70-81.

8.   EC 1.14.16.1. http://www.chem.qmul.ac.uk/iubmb/enzyme/EC1/14/16/1.html. Accessed February 27, 2007.

9.   Seashore MR. Tetrahydrobiopterin and Dietary Restriction in Mild Phenylketonuria. *N Engl J Med.* 2002;347(26):2094-2095.

10.   Muntau AC, Roschinger W, Habich M, et al. Tetrahydrobiopterin as an Alternative Treatment for Mild Phenylketonuria. *N Engl J Med.* 2002;347(26):2122-2132.

11.   Kure S, Hou D-C, Ohura T, et al. Tetrahydrobiopterin-responsive phenylalanine hydroxylase deficiency. *The Journal of Pediatrics.* 1999;135(3):375-378.

12.   Watson JD, Crick FH. Molecular structure of nucleic acids; a structure for deoxyribose nucleic acid. *Nature.* Apr 25 1953;171(4356):737-738.

13.   Wright R. James Watson & Francis Crick. web page] http://www.time.com/time/time100/scientist/profile/watsoncrick.html. Accessed December 11, 2005.

14. Attia J, Ioannidis JPA, Thakkinstian A, et al. How to Use an Article About Genetic Association: C: What Are the Results and Will They Help Me in Caring for My Patients? *JAMA.* 2009;301(3):304-308.

15. Attia J, Ioannidis JPA, Thakkinstian A, et al. How to Use an Article About Genetic Association: B: Are the Results of the Study Valid? *JAMA.* 2009;301(2):191-197.

16. Attia J, Ioannidis JPA, Thakkinstian A, et al. How to Use an Article About Genetic Association: A: Background Concepts. *JAMA.* 2009;301(1):74-81.

17. McGuire AL, Burke W. An Unwelcome Side Effect of Direct-to-Consumer Personal Genome Testing: Raiding the Medical Commons. *JAMA.* 2008;300(22):2669-2671.

18. Initial sequencing and analysis of the human genome. *Nature.* 2001;409(6822):860-921.

19. Banks RE, Dunn MJ, Hochstrasser DF, et al. Proteomics: new perspectives, new biomedical opportunities. *Lancet.* Nov 18 2000;356(9243):1749-1756.

20. Rock CL, Lampe JW, Patterson RE. Nutrition, Genetics, and Risks of Cancer. *Annual Review of Public Health.* 2000;21(1):47-64.

21. van Meurs JBJ, Dhonukshe-Rutten RAM, Pluijm SMF, et al. Homocysteine Levels and the Risk of Osteoporotic Fracture. *N Engl J Med.* 2004;350(20):2033-2041.

22. Rimm EB, Willett WC, Hu FB, et al. Folate and Vitamin B6 From Diet and Supplements in Relation to Risk of Coronary Heart Disease Among Women. *JAMA.* 1998;279(5):359-364.

23. Kim Y-I. Nutritional Epigenetics: Impact of Folate Deficiency on DNA Methylation and Colon Cancer Susceptibility. *J. Nutr.* 2005;135(11):2703-2709.

24. Klerk M, Verhoef P, Clarke R, Blom HJ, Kok FJ, Schouten EG. MTHFR 677C-->T polymorphism and risk of coronary heart disease: a meta-analysis. *Jama.* Oct 23-30 2002;288(16):2023-2031.

25. Brown AA, Hu FB. Dietary modulation of endothelial function: implications for cardiovascular disease. *Am J Clin Nutr.* 2001;73(4):673-686.

26. Ravaglia G, Forti P, Maioli F, et al. Homocysteine and cognitive function in healthy elderly community dwellers in Italy. *Am J Clin Nutr.* 2003;77(3):668-673.

27. Seshadri S, Beiser A, Selhub J, et al. Plasma homocysteine as a risk factor for dementia and Alzheimer's disease. *N Engl J Med.* Feb 14 2002;346(7):476-483.

28. Welch GN, Loscalzo J. Homocysteine and Atherothrombosis. *N Engl J Med.* 1998;338(15):1042-1050.

29. Malinow MR, Nieto FJ, Kruger WD, et al. The Effects of Folic Acid Supplementation on Plasma Total Homocysteine Are Modulated by Multivitamin Use and Methylenetetrahydrofolate Reductase Genotypes. *Arterioscler Thromb Vasc Biol.* 1997;17(6):1157-1162.

30. den Heijer M, Brouwer IA, Bos GMJ, et al. Vitamin Supplementation Reduces Blood Homocysteine Levels : A Controlled Trial in Patients With Venous Thrombosis and Healthy Volunteers. *Arterioscler Thromb Vasc Biol.* 1998;18(3):356-361.

31. Bressler R. Herb-drug interactions: interactions between Ginkgo biloba and prescription medications. *Geriatrics.* Apr 2005;60(4):30-33.

32. Bressler R, Bahl JJ. Principles of drug therapy for the elderly patient. *Mayo Clin Proc.* Dec 2003;78(12):1564-1577.

33. Wilkinson GW. Pharmacokinetics: The dynamics of drug absorption, distribution, and elimination. In: Goodman AG, Hardman JG, Limbird LE, eds. *The Pharmacological Basis of Therapeutics.* 10th ed. New York, NY: McGraw-Hill Book Co.; 2001:3-29.

34. Lai C, Shields PG. The Role of Interindividual Variation in Human Carcinogenesis. *J. Nutr.* 1999;129(2):552S-555S.

35. Carnell DM, Smith RE, Daley FM, et al. Target validation of cytochrome P450 CYP1B1 in prostate carcinoma with protein expression in associated hyperplastic and premalignant tissue. *International Journal of Radiation Oncology*Biology*Physics.* 2004;58(2):500-509.

36. Cheung YL, Kerr AC, McFadyen MC, Melvin WT, Murray GI. Differential expression of CYP1A1, CYP1A2, CYP1B1 in human kidney tumours. *Cancer Lett.* May 24 1999;139(2):199-205.

37. McFadyen MC, Breeman S, Payne S, et al. Immunohistochemical localization of cytochrome P450 CYP1B1 in breast cancer with monoclonal antibodies specific for CYP1B1. *J Histochem Cytochem.* Nov 1999;47(11):1457-1464.

38. McFadyen MC, McLeod HL, Jackson FC, Melvin WT, Doehmer J, Murray GI. Cytochrome P450 CYP1B1 protein expression: a novel mechanism of anticancer drug resistance. *Biochem Pharmacol.* Jul 15 2001;62(2):207-212.

39. Murray GI, Taylor MC, McFadyen MC, et al. Tumor-specific expression of cytochrome P450 CYP1B1. *Cancer Res.* Jul 15 1997;57(14):3026-3031.

40. Muti P, Bradlow HL, Micheli A, et al. Estrogen metabolism and risk of breast cancer: a prospective study of the 2:16alpha-hydroxyestrone ratio in premenopausal and postmenopausal women. *Epidemiology.* Nov 2000;11(6):635-640.

41. Dalessandri KM, Firestone GL, Fitch MD, Bradlow HL, Bjeldanes LF. Pilot Study: Effect of 3,3'-Diindolylmethane Supplements on Urinary Hormone Metabolites in Postmenopausal Women With a History of Early-Stage Breast Cancer. *Nutrition and Cancer.* 2004;50(2):161-167.

42. Gershon M. *The Second Brain: A Groundbreaking New Understanding of Nervous Disorders of the Stomach and Intestine.* New York: Harper Paperbacks; 1999.

43. Saavedra JM, Tschernia A. Human studies with probiotics and prebiotics: clinical implications. *Br J Nutr.* May 2002;87 Suppl 2:S241-246.

44. Bengmark S. Immunonutrition: role of biosurfactants, fiber, and probiotic bacteria. *Nutrition.* Jul-Aug 1998;14(7-8):585-594.

45. Kirjavainen PV, Gibson GR. Healthy gut microflora and allergy: factors influencing development of the microbiota. *Ann Med.* Aug 1999;31(4):288-292.

46. Barbeau WE. Interactions between dietary proteins and the human system: implications for oral tolerance and food-related diseases. *Adv Exp Med Biol.* 1997;415:183-193.

47. Stanley S. Oral tolerance of food. *Curr Allergy Asthma Rep.* Jan 2002;2(1):73-77.

48. Schneeman BO. Gastrointestinal physiology and functions. *Br J Nutr.* Nov 2002;88 Suppl 2:S159-163.

49. Hurwitz A, Brady DA, Schaal SE, Samloff IM, Dedon J, Ruhl CE. Gastric acidity in older adults. *Jama.* Aug 27 1997;278(8):659-662.

50. Kassarjian Z, Russell RM. Hypochlorhydria: A Factor in Nutrition. *Annual Review of Nutrition.* 1989;9(1):271-285.

51. Wood RJ, Suter PM, Russell RM. Mineral requirements of elderly people. *Am J Clin Nutr.* 1995;62(3):493-505.

52. Baik HW, Russell RM. Vitamin B12 deficiency in the elderly. *Annu Rev Nutr.* 1999;19:357-377.

53. Prousky JE. Cobalamin deficiency in elderly patients. *CMAJ.* 2005;172(4):450-a-451.

54. Sturniolo GC, Montino MC, Rossetto L, et al. Inhibition of gastric acid secretion reduces zinc absorption in man. *J Am Coll Nutr.* Aug 1991;10(4):372-375.

55. Kelly GS. Hydrochloric Acid: Physiological Functions and Clinical Implications. *Alt Med Rev.* 1997;2(2):116-127.

56. Sharp GS. The diagnosis and treatment of achlorhydria; preliminary report of new simplified methods. *West J Surg Obstet Gynecol.* Jul 1953;61(7):353-360.

57. Yang YX, Lewis JD, Epstein S, Metz DC. Long-term proton pump inhibitor therapy and risk of hip fracture. *JAMA.* 2006;296(24):2947-2953.

58. Martinsen TC, Bergh K, Waldum HL. Gastric juice: a barrier against infectious diseases. *Basic Clin Pharmacol Toxicol.* Feb 2005;96(2):94-102.

59. Hongo M, Ishimori A, Nagasaki A, Sato T. Effect of duodenal acidification on the lower esophageal sphincter pressure in the dog with special reference to related gastrointestinal hormones. *Tohoku J Exp Med.* Jul 1980;131(3):215-219.

60. Wright JV. *Dr. Wright's Guide to Healing with Nutrition.* New Canaan, CT: Keats Publishing; 1990.

61. Tomohiko S, Masaki I, Nobue H, Yoko H, Masuo N, Susumu T. Gastric Acid Normosecretion Is Not Essential in the Pathogenesis of Mild Erosive Gastroesophageal Reflux Disease in Relation to Helicobacter pylori Status. *Digestive Diseases and Sciences.* 2004;V49(5):787-794.

62. Bralley J, Lord R. Chapter 4: Amino Acids. *Laboratory Evaluations in Molecular Medicine: Nutrients, Toxicants, and Cell Regulators.* Norcross, GA: The Institute for Advances in Molecular Medicine; 2001:75-131.

63. Simon GL, Gorbach SL. Intestinal flora in health and disease. *Gastroenterology.* Jan 1984;86(1):174-193.

64. Guarner F, Malagelada J-R. Gut flora in health and disease. *The Lancet.* 2003;361(9356):512-519.

65. Bengmark S. Ecological control of the gastrointestinal tract. The role of probiotic flora. *Gut.* Jan 1998;42(1):2-7.

66. Laheij RJF, Sturkenboom MCJM, Hassing R-J, Dieleman J, Stricker BHC, Jansen JBMJ. Risk of Community-Acquired Pneumonia and Use of Gastric Acid-Suppressive Drugs. *JAMA.* 2004;292(16):1955-1960.

67. Bralley J, Lord R. *Laboratory Evaluations in Molecular Medicine: Nutrients, Toxicants, and Cell Regulators.* Norcross, GA: The Institute for Advances in Molecular Medicine; 2001.

68. Urita Y, Sugimoto M, Hike K, et al. High incidence of fermentation in the digestive tract in patients with reflux oesophagitis. *Eur J Gastroenterol Hepatol.* May 2006;18(5):531-535.

69. Santos J, Bayarri C, Saperas E, et al. Characterisation of immune mediator release during the immediate response to segmental mucosal challenge in the jejunum of patients with food allergy. *Gut.* 1999;45(4):553-558.

70. Rodrigo L. Celiac disease. *World J Gastroenterol.* Nov 7 2006;12(41):6585-6593.

71. Hernandez L, Green PH. Extraintestinal manifestations of celiac disease. *Curr Gastroenterol Rep.* Oct 2006;8(5):383-389.

72. Hvatum M, Kanerud L, Hallgren R, Brandtzaeg P. The gut-joint axis: cross reactive food antibodies in rheumatoid arthritis. *Gut.* 2006;55(9):1240-1247.

73. Zar S, Kumar D, Benson MJ. Food hypersensitivity and irritable bowel syndrome. *Alimentary Pharmacology & Therapeutics.* 2001;15(4):439-449.

74. Rowntree S, Platts-Mills TA, Cogswell JJ, Mitchell EB. A subclass IgG4-specific antigen-binding radioimmunoassay (RIA): comparison between IgG and IgG4 antibodies to food and inhaled antigens in adult atopic dermatitis after desensitization treatment and during development of antibody responses in children. *J Allergy Clin Immunol.* Oct 1987;80(4):622-630.

75. Calkhoven PG, Aalbers M, Koshte VL, et al. Relationship between IgG1 and IgG4 antibodies to foods and the development of IgE antibodies to inhalant allergens. II. Increased levels of IgG antibodies to foods in children who subsequently develop IgE antibodies to inhalant allergens. *Clin Exp Allergy.* Jan 1991;21(1):99-107.

76. McKinnon RA, McManus ME. Localization of cytochromes P450 in human tissues: implications for chemical toxicity. *Pathology.* May 1996;28(2):148-155.

77. McKinnon RA, Burgess WM, Hall PM, Roberts-Thomson SJ, Gonzalez FJ, McManus ME. Characterisation of CYP3A gene subfamily expression in human gastrointestinal tissues. *Gut.* Feb 1995;36(2):259-267.

78. Johnstone RW, Ruefli AA, Smyth MJ. Multiple physiological functions for multidrug transporter P-glycoprotein? *Trends in Biochemical Sciences.* 2000/1/1 2000;25(1):1-6.

79. Izzo AA. Herb-drug interactions: an overview of the clinical evidence. *Fundamental and Clinical Pharmacology.* 2005;19(1):1-16.

80. Scheline RR. Metabolism of foreign compounds by gastrointestinal microorganisms. *Pharmacol Rev.* Dec 1973;25(4):451-523.

81. Cummings JH. Fermentation in the human large intestine: evidence and implications for health. *Lancet.* May 28 1983;1(8335):1206-1209.

82. Turner EH, Matthews AM, Linardatos E, Tell RA, Rosenthal R. Selective Publication of Antidepressant Trials and Its Influence on Apparent Efficacy. *N Engl J Med.* 2008;358(3):252-260.

83. Woloshin S, Schwartz LM. Giving Legs to Restless Legs: A Case Study of How the Media Helps Make People Sick. *PLoS Medicine.* 2006;3(4):e170.

84. Committee on N. Cholesterol in Childhood. *Pediatrics.* 1998;101(1):141-147.

85. Boustani M, Hall KS, Lane KA, et al. The Association Between Cognition and Histamine-2 Receptor Antagonists in African Americans. *Journal of the American Geriatrics Society.* 2007;55(8):1248-1253.

86. FDA Issues Safety Alert on Avandia. [web page]. May 21, 2007; http://www.fda.gov/bbs/topics/NEWS/2007/NEW01636.html. Accessed August 1, 2007.

87. Camilleri M, Choi MG. Review article: irritable bowel syndrome. *Aliment Pharmacol Ther.* Feb 1997;11(1):3-15.

88. Drossman DA, Li Z, Andruzzi E, et al. U.S. householder survey of functional gastrointestinal disorders. Prevalence, sociodemography, and health impact. *Dig Dis Sci.* Sep 1993;38(9):1569-1580.

89. Talley NJ, Zinsmeister AR, Van Dyke C, Melton LJ, 3rd. Epidemiology of colonic symptoms and the irritable bowel syndrome. *Gastroenterology.* Oct 1991;101(4):927-934.

90. Leong SA, Barghout V, Birnbaum HG, et al. The economic consequences of irritable bowel syndrome: a US employer perspective. *Arch Intern Med.* Apr 28 2003;163(8):929-935.

91. Talley NJ, Gabriel SE, Harmsen WS, Zinsmeister AR, Evans RW. Medical costs in community subjects with irritable bowel syndrome. *Gastroenterology.* Dec 1995;109(6):1736-1741.

92. Whitehead WE, Cheskin LJ, Heller BR, et al. Evidence for exacerbation of irritable bowel syndrome during menses. *Gastroenterology.* Jun 1990;98(6):1485-1489.

93. Burns DG. The risk of abdominal surgery in irritable bowel syndrome (abstr.). *S Afr Med J.* Jul 19 1986;70(2):91.

94. Martin R, Barron JJ, Zacker C. Irritable bowel syndrome: toward a cost-effective management approach. *Am J Manag Care.* Jul 2001;7(8 Suppl):S268-275.

95. Everhart JE, Renault PF. Irritable bowel syndrome in office-based practice in the United States. *Gastroenterology.* Apr 1991;100(4):998-1005.

96. Sandler RS. Epidemiology of irritable bowel syndrome in the United States. *Gastroenterology.* Aug 1990;99(2):409-415.

97. Keefer L, Blanchard EB. The effects of relaxation response meditation on the symptoms of irritable bowel syndrome: results of a controlled treatment study. *Behav Res Ther.* Jul 2001;39(7):801-811.

98. Park MI, Camilleri M. Is there a role of food allergy in irritable bowel syndrome and functional dyspepsia? A systematic review. *Neurogastroenterol Motil.* Aug 2006;18(8):595-607.

99. O'Mahony L, McCarthy J, Kelly P, et al. Lactobacillus and bifidobacterium in irritable bowel syndrome: Symptom responses and relationship to cytokine profiles. *Gastroenterology.* 2005;128(3):541-551.

100. Kajander K, Hatakka K, Poussa T, Farkkila M, Korpela R. A probiotic mixture alleviates symptoms in irritable bowel syndrome patients: a controlled 6-month intervention. *Aliment Pharmacol Ther.* Sep 1 2005;22(5):387-394.

101. Kline RM, Kline JJ, Di Palma J, Barbero GJ. Enteric-coated, pH-dependent peppermint oil capsules for the treatment of irritable bowel syndrome in children. *J Pediatr.* Jan 2001;138(1):125-128.

102. Iwamoto I, Kosha S, Noguchi S-i, et al. A longitudinal study of the effect of vitamin K2 on bone mineral density in postmenopausal women a comparative study with vitamin D3 and estrogen-progestin therapy. *Maturitas.* 1999;31(2):161-164.

103. Purwosunu Y, Muharram, Rachman IA, Reksoprodjo S, Sekizawa A. Vitamin K2 treatment for postmenopausal osteoporosis in Indonesia. *J Obstet Gynaecol Res.* Apr 2006;32(2):230-234.

104. Yasui T, Miyatani Y, Tomita J, et al. Effect of vitamin K2 treatment on carboxylation of osteocalcin in early postmenopausal women. *Gynecological Endocrinology.* 2006;22(8):455-459.

105. Ushiroyama T, Ikeda A, Ueki M. Effect of continuous combined therapy with vitamin K2 and vitamin D3 on bone mineral density and coagulofibrinolysis function in postmenopausal women. *Maturitas.* 2002;41(3):211-221.

106. Shiraki M, Shiraki Y, Aoki C, Miura M. Vitamin K2 (Menatetrenone) Effectively Prevents Fractures and Sustains Lumbar Bone Mineral Density in Osteoporosis. *Journal of Bone and Mineral Research.* 2000;15(3):515-522.

107. Asakura H, Myou S, Ontachi Y, et al. Vitamin K administration to elderly patients with osteoporosis induces no hemostatic activation, even in those with suspected vitamin K deficiency. *Osteoporos Int.* Dec 2001;12(12):996-1000.

108. Ronden JE, Groenen-van Dooren MMCL, Hornstra G, Vermeer C. Modulation of arterial thrombosis tendency in rats by vitamin K and its side chains. *Atherosclerosis.* 1997;132(1):61-67.

109. Cockayne S, Adamson J, Lanham-New S, Shearer MJ, Gilbody S, Torgerson DJ. Vitamin K and the Prevention of Fractures: Systematic Review and Meta-analysis of Randomized Controlled Trials. *Arch Intern Med.* 2006;166(12):1256-1261.

110. Plaza SM, Lamson DW. Vitamin K2 in bone metabolism and osteoporosis. *Altern Med Rev.* Mar 2005;10(1):24-35.

111. Schurgers LJ, Teunissen KJF, Hamulyak K, Knapen MHJ, Vik H, Vermeer C. Vitamin K-containing dietary supplements: comparison of synthetic vitamin K1 and natto-derived menaquinone-7. *Blood.* 2007;109(8):3279-3283.

112. Rosenberg IH. Summary comments. *Am J Clin Nutr.* 1989;50(5):1231-1233.

113. Doherty TJ. Invited Review: Aging and sarcopenia. *J Appl Physiol*. 2003;95(4):1717-1727.

114. Solerte SB, Gazzaruso C, Bonacasa R, et al. Nutritional Supplements with Oral Amino Acid Mixtures Increases Whole-Body Lean Mass and Insulin Sensitivity in Elderly Subjects with Sarcopenia. *The American Journal of Cardiology*. 2008;101(11, Supplement 1):S69-S77.

115. Bales CW, Ritchie CS. Sarcopenia, Weight Loss, and Nutritional Frailty in the Elderly. *Annual Review of Nutrition*. 2002;22(1):309-323.

116. Kamel HK. Sarcopenia and aging. *Nutrition Reviews*. 2003;61(5 part 1):157-167.

117. Looker AC, Orwoll ES, Johnston CC, et al. Prevalence of Low Femoral Bone Density in Older U.S. Adults from NHANES III. *Journal of Bone and Mineral Research*. 1997;12(11):1761-1768.

118. Hampton T. Experts Urge Early Investment in Bone Health. *JAMA*. February 18, 2004 2004;291(7):811-812.

119. Burge R, Dawson-Hughes B, Solomon DH, Wong JB, King A, Tosteson A. Incidence and Economic Burden of Osteoporosis-Related Fractures in the United States, 2005-2025. *Journal of Bone and Mineral Research*. 2007;22(3):465-475.

120. Management of osteoporosis in postmenopausal women: 2006 position statement of The North American Menopause Society. *Menopause*. May-Jun 2006;13(3):340-367; quiz 368-349.

121. Old JL, Calvert M. Vertebral compression fractures in the elderly. *Am Fam Physician*. Jan 1 2004;69(1):111-116.

122. Cooper C, Atkinson EJ, Jacobsen SJ, O'Fallon WM, Melton LJ, 3rd. Population-based study of survival after osteoporotic fractures. *Am J Epidemiol*. May 1 1993;137(9):1001-1005.

123. Melton LJ, 3rd, Chrischilles EA, Cooper C, Lane AW, Riggs BL. Perspective. How many women have osteoporosis? [abstract]. *J Bone Miner Res*. Sep 1992;7(9):1005-1010.

124. Gregg EW, Cauley JA, Seeley DG, Ensrud KE, Bauer DC. Physical activity and osteoporotic fracture risk in older women. Study of Osteoporotic Fractures Research Group. *Ann Intern Med*. Jul 15 1998;129(2):81-88.

125. Bliuc D, Nguyen ND, Milch VE, Nguyen TV, Eisman JA, Center JR. Mortality Risk Associated With Low-Trauma Osteoporotic Fracture and Subsequent Fracture in Men and Women. *JAMA*. 2009;301(5):513-521.

126. Czerwinski E, Badurski JE, Marcinowska-Suchowierska E, Osieleniec J. Current understanding of osteoporosis according to the position of the World Health Organization (WHO) and International Osteoporosis Foundation. *Ortop Traumatol Rehabil*. Jul-Aug 2007;9(4):337-356.

127. Siris ES, Chen Y-T, Abbott TA, et al. Bone Mineral Density Thresholds for Pharmacological Intervention to Prevent Fractures. *Arch Intern Med*. 2004;164(10):1108-1112.

128. Kanis JA, Johnell O, Oden A, De Laet C, Jonsson B, Dawson A. Ten-year risk of osteoporotic fracture and the effect of risk factors on screening strategies. *Bone*. 2002;30(1):251-258.

129. Schuit SC, van der Klift M, Weel AE, et al. Fracture incidence and association with bone mineral density in elderly men and women: the Rotterdam Study. *Bone*. Jan 2004;34(1):195-202.

130. Krane S, Holick M. Metabolic Bone Disease: Osteoporosis. In: Isselbacher K, Brunwald E, Wilson J, eds. *Harrison's Principles of Internal Medicine*. New York: McGraw Hill, Inc.; 1994:2172-2176.

131. Murray MT, Pizzorno JE. Osteoporosis. *Textbook of Natural Medicine*. 2nd ed: Churchill Livingstone; 1999:1453-1462.

132. McGarry KA, Kiel DP. Postmenopausal osteoporosis. Strategies for preventing bone loss, avoiding fracture. *Postgrad Med*. Sep 1 2000;108(3):79-82, 85-78, 91.

133. Sunyer T, Lewis J, Collin-Osdoby P, Osdoby P. Estrogen's bone-protective effects may involve differential IL-1 receptor regulation in human osteoclast-like cells. *J. Clin. Invest*. May 15, 1999 1999;103(10):1409-1418.

134. Knutson D, Greenberg G, Cronau H. Management of crohn's disease--a practical approach. *Am Fam Physician*. 2003;68:707-714.

135. Lydeking-Olsen E, Beck-Jensen JE, Setchell KD, Holm-Jensen T. Soymilk or progesterone for prevention of bone loss: a 2 year randomized, placebo-controlled trial. *Eur J Nutr*. Aug 2004;43(4):246-257.

136. Yun AJ, Lee PY. Maldaptation of the link between inflammation and bone turnover may be a key determinant of osteoporosis. *Medical Hypotheses.* 2004;63(3):532-537.

137. Van Staa TP, Leufkens HGM, Abenhaim L, Zhang B, Cooper C. Use of oral corticosteroids and risk of fractures. *J Bone Miner Res.* June 2000;15(6):993-1000.

138. Van Staa TP, Laan RF, Barton IP, Cohen S, Reid DM, Cooper C. Bone density threshold and other predictors of vertebral fracture in patients receiving oral glucocorticoid therapy. *Arthritis Rheum.* Nov 2003;48(11):3224-3229.

139. Hara K, Kobayashi M, Akiyama Y. Vitamin K2 (menatetrenone) inhibits bone loss induced by prednisolone partly through enhancement of bone formation in rats. *Bone.* Nov 2002;31(5):575-581.

140. Yonemura K, Fukasawa H, Fujigaki Y, Hishida A. Protective effect of vitamins K2 and D3 on prednisolone-induced loss of bone mineral density in the lumbar spine. *Am J Kidney Dis.* Jan 2004;43(1):53-60.

141. Dennison E, Hindmarsh P, Fall C, et al. Profiles of Endogenous Circulating Cortisol and Bone Mineral Density in Healthy Elderly Men. *J Clin Endocrinol Metab.* September 1, 1999 1999;84(9):3058-3063.

142. Wang H, Zhu G, Shi Y, et al. Influence of environmental cadmium exposure on forearm bone density. *J Bone Miner Res.* Mar 2003;18(3):553-560.

143. Alfven T, Elinder CG, Carlsson MD, et al. Low-level cadmium exposure and osteoporosis. *J Bone Miner Res.* Aug 2000;15(8):1579-1586.

144. Kazantzis G. Cadmium, osteoporosis and calcium metabolism. *Biometals.* Oct 2004;17(5):493-498.

145. Uriu K, Morimoto I, Kai K, et al. Uncoupling between bone formation and resorption in ovariectomized rats with chronic cadmium exposure. *Toxicol Appl Pharmacol.* May 1 2000;164(3):264-272.

146. Maurer M, Riesen W, Muser J, Hulter HN, Krapf R. Neutralization of Western diet inhibits bone resorption independently of K intake and reduces cortisol secretion in humans. *Am J Physiol Renal Physiol.* January 1, 2003 2003;284(1):F32-40.

147. McLean RR, Jacques PF, Selhub J, et al. Homocysteine as a Predictive Factor for Hip Fracture in Older Persons. *N Engl J Med.* May 13, 2004 2004;350(20):2042-2049.

148. Miller AL. Cardiovascular Disease--Toward a Unified Approach. *Alt Med Rev.* 1996;1(3):132-147.

149. Upchurch GR, Jr., Welch GN, Fabian AJ, et al. Homocyst(e)ine decreases bioavailable nitric oxide by a mechanism involving glutathione peroxidase. *J Biol Chem.* Jul 4 1997;272(27):17012-17017.

150. Nygard O, Nordrehaug JE, Refsum H, Ueland PM, Farstad M, Vollset SE. Plasma Homocysteine Levels and Mortality in Patients with Coronary Artery Disease. *N Engl J Med.* July 24, 1997 1997;337(4):230-237.

151. Harris SS, Dawson-Hughes B. Caffeine and bone loss in healthy postmenopausal women. *Am J Clin Nutr.* Oct 1994;60(4):573-578.

152. Heaney RP. Effects of caffeine on bone and the calcium economy. *Food Chem Toxicol.* Sep 2002;40(9):1263-1270.

153. Meyer HE, Pedersen JI, Loken EB, Tverdal A. Dietary factors and the incidence of hip fracture in middle-aged Norwegians. A prospective study. *Am J Epidemiol.* Jan 15 1997;145(2):117-123.

154. Prince RL, Smith M, Dick IM, et al. Prevention of postmenopausal osteoporosis. A comparative study of exercise, calcium supplementation, and hormone-replacement therapy. *N Engl J Med.* Oct 24 1991;325(17):1189-1195.

155. Thomas TN. Lifestyle risk factors for osteoporosis. *Medsurg Nurs.* Oct 1997;6(5):275-277, 287.

156. Bonaiuti D, Shea B, Iovine R, et al. Exercise for preventing and treating osteoporosis in postmenopausal women. *Cochrane Database Syst Rev.* 2002(3):CD000333.

157. Wolff I, van Croonenborg JJ, Kemper HC, Kostense PJ, Twisk JW. The effect of exercise training programs on bone mass: a meta-analysis of published controlled trials in pre- and postmenopausal women. *Osteoporos Int.* 1999;9(1):1-12.

158. Macera CA. Exercise and risk of hip fracture in postmenopausal women. *Clin J Sport Med.* Mar 2004;14(2):103-104.

159. Englund U, Littbrand H, Sondell A, Pettersson U, Bucht G. A 1-year combined weight-bearing training program is beneficial for bone mineral density and neuromuscular function in older women. *Osteoporosis International.* 2005;16(9):1117-1123.

160. NIH Consensus Development Panel on Osteoporosis Prevention, Diagnosis, and Therapy, March 7-29, 2000: highlights of the conference. *South Med J.* 2001;94(6):569-573.

161. Robertson MC, Campbell AJ, Gardner MM, Devlin N. Preventing injuries in older people by preventing falls: a meta-analysis of individual-level data. *J Am Geriatr Soc.* 2002;50(5):905-911.

162. Clinical Management Guidelines for Obstetrician-Gynecologists. Number 50, January 2003(Replaces Committee Opinion Number 270, March 2002 and Educational Bulletin Number 246, April 1998): Osteoporosis. *Obstet Gynecol.* 2004;103(1):203-216.

163. Maggio D, Barabani M, Pierandrei M, et al. Marked Decrease in Plasma Antioxidants in Aged Osteoporotic Women: Results of a Cross-Sectional Study. *J Clin Endocrinol Metab.* April 1, 2003 2003;88(4):1523-1527.

164. Kaptoge S, Benevolenskaya LI, Bhalla AK, et al. Low BMD is less predictive than reported falls for future limb fractures in women across Europe: results from the European Prospective Osteoporosis Study. *Bone.* 2005;36(3):387-398.

165. Green AD, Colon-Emeric CS, Bastian L, Drake MT, Lyles KW. Does This Woman Have Osteoporosis? *JAMA.* 2004;292(23):2890-2900.

166. Siminoski K, Jiang G, Adachi JD, et al. Accuracy of height loss during prospective monitoring for detection of incident vertebral fractures. *Osteoporosis International.* 2005;16(4):403-410.

167. Black DM, Cummings SR, Karpf DB, et al. Randomised trial of effect of alendronate on risk of fracture in women with existing vertebral fractures. Fracture Intervention Trial Research Group. *Lancet.* 1996;348(9041):1535-1541.

168. Reginster J, Minne HW, Sorensen OH, et al. Randomized trial of the effects of risedronate on vertebral fractures in women with established postmenopausal osteoporosis. Vertebral Efficacy with Risedronate Therapy (VERT) Study Group. *Osteoporos Int.* 2000;11(1):83-91.

169. Ettinger B, Black DM, Mitlak BH, et al. Reduction of vertebral fracture risk in postmenopausal women with osteoporosis treated with raloxifene: results from a 3-year

randomized clinical trial. Multiple Outcomes of Raloxifene Evaluation (MORE) Investigators. *Jama.* 1999;282(7):637-645.

170. Neer RM, Arnaud CD, Zanchetta JR, et al. Effect of parathyroid hormone (1-34) on fractures and bone mineral density in postmenopausal women with osteoporosis. *N Engl J Med.* 2001;344(19):1434-1441.

171. Sarkar S, Mitlak BH, Wong M, Stock JL, Black DM, Harper KD. Relationships Between Bone Mineral Density and Incident Vertebral Fracture Risk with Raloxifene Therapy. *Journal of Bone and Mineral Research.* 2002;17(1):1-10.

172. Sarkar S, Reginster J-Y, Crans GG, Diez-Perez A, Pinette KV, Delmas PD. Relationship Between Changes in Biochemical Markers of Bone Turnover and BMD to Predict Vertebral Fracture Risk. *Journal of Bone and Mineral Research.* 2004;19(3):394-401.

173. Cummings SR, Karpf DB, Harris F, et al. Improvement in spine bone density and reduction in risk of vertebral fractures during treatment with antiresorptive drugs. *Am J Med.* Mar 2002;112(4):281-289.

174. Li Z, Meredith MP, Hoseyni MS. A method to assess the proportion of treatment effect explained by a surrogate endpoint. *Stat Med.* Nov 15 2001;20(21):3175-3188.

175. Neviaser AS, Lane JM, Lenart BA, Edobor-Osula F, Lorich DG. Low-energy femoral shaft fractures associated with alendronate use. *J Orthop Trauma.* May-Jun 2008;22(5):346-350.

176. Goh SK, Yang KY, Koh JSB, et al. Subtrochanteric insufficiency fractures in patients on alendronate therapy: A CAUTION. *J Bone Joint Surg Br.* 2007;89-B(3):349-353.

177. Odvina CV, Zerwekh JE, Rao DS, Maalouf N, Gottschalk FA, Pak CYC. Severely Suppressed Bone Turnover: A Potential Complication of Alendronate Therapy. *J Clin Endocrinol Metab.* 2005;90(3):1294-1301.

178. Braam LA, Knapen MH, Geusens P, et al. Vitamin K1 supplementation retards bone loss in postmenopausal women between 50 and 60 years of age. *Calcif Tissue Int.* Jul 2003;73(1):21-26.

179. Grant AM, Avenell A, Campbell MK, et al. Oral vitamin D3 and calcium for secondary prevention of low-trauma fractures in elderly people (Randomised Evaluation of Calcium Or vitamin D, RECORD): a randomised placebo-controlled trial. *Lancet.* May 7-13 2005;365(9471):1621-1628.

180. Larsen ER, Mosekilde L, Foldspang A. Vitamin D and Calcium Supplementation Prevents Osteoporotic Fractures in Elderly Community Dwelling Residents: A Pragmatic Population-Based 3-Year Intervention Study. *Journal of Bone and Mineral Research.* 2004;19(3):370-378.

181. Meier C, Woitge HW, Witte K, Lemmer B, Seibel MJ. Supplementation With Oral Vitamin D3 and Calcium During Winter Prevents Seasonal Bone Loss: A Randomized Controlled Open-Label Prospective Trial. *Journal of Bone and Mineral Research.* 2004;19(8):1221-1230.

182. Conly J, Stein K. Reduction of vitamin K2 concentrations in human liver associated with the use of broad spectrum antimicrobials. *Clin Invest Med.* Dec 1994;17(6):531-539.

183. Ferland G, Sadowski JA, O'Brien ME. Dietary induced subclinical vitamin K deficiency in normal human subjects. *J Clin Invest.* Apr 1993;91(4):1761-1768.

184. Hodges SJ, Pilkington MJ, Shearer MJ, Bitensky L, Chayen J. Age-related changes in the circulating levels of congeners of vitamin K2, menaquinone-7 and menaquinone-8. *Clin Sci (Lond).* Jan 1990;78(1):63-66.

185. Sontakke AN, Tare RS. A duality in the roles of reactive oxygen species with respect to bone metabolism. *Clinica Chimica Acta.* 2002/4 2002;318(1-2):145-148.

186. Hall SL, Greendale GA. The relation of dietary vitamin C intake to bone mineral density: results from the PEPI study. *Calcif Tissue Int.* Oct 1998;63(3):183-189.

187. Wang MC, Luz Villa M, Marcus R, Kelsey JL. Associations of vitamin C, calcium and protein with bone mass in postmenopausal Mexican American women. *Osteoporos Int.* 1997;7(6):533-538.

188. Melhus H, Michaelsson K, Holmberg L, Wolk A, Ljunghall S. Smoking, antioxidant vitamins, and the risk of hip fracture. *J Bone Miner Res.* Feb 1999;14(1):129-135.

189. Lean JM, Davies JT, Fuller K, et al. A crucial role for thiol antioxidants in estrogen-deficiency bone loss. *J Clin Invest.* Sep 2003;112(6):915-923.

190. Cashman KD. Calcium intake, calcium bioavailability and bone health. *Br J Nutr.* May 2002;87 Suppl 2:S169-177.

191. Heaney RP. Long-latency deficiency disease: insights from calcium and vitamin D. *Am J Clin Nutr.* November 1, 2003 2003;78(5):912-919.

192. Tucker KL, Hannan MT, Chen H, Cupples LA, Wilson PW, Kiel DP. Potassium, magnesium, and fruit and vegetable intakes are associated with greater bone mineral density in elderly men and women. *Am J Clin Nutr.* April 1, 1999 1999;69(4):727-736.

193. Szulc P, Arlot M, Chapuy MC, Duboeuf F, Meunier PJ, Delmas PD. Serum undercarboxylated osteocalcin correlates with hip bone mineral density in elderly women. *J Bone Miner Res.* 1994;9:1591-1595.

194. Hyun TH, Barrett-Connor E, Milne DB. Zinc intakes and plasma concentrations in men with osteoporosis: the Rancho Bernardo Study. *Am J Clin Nutr.* September 1, 2004 2004;80(3):715-721.

195. Lowe NM, Fraser WD, Jackson MJ. Is there a potential therapeutic value of copper and zinc for osteoporosis? *Proc Nutr Soc.* May 2002;61(2):181-185.

196. Marie PJ, Hott M, Modrowski D, et al. An uncoupling agent containing strontium prevents bone loss by depressing bone resorption and maintaining bone formation in estrogen-deficient rats. *J Bone Miner Res.* May 1993;8(5):607-615.

197. Caverzasio J. Strontium ranelate promotes osteoblastic cell replication through at least two different mechanisms. *Bone.* 2008;42(6):1131-1136.

198. Meunier PJ, Slosman DO, Delmas PD, et al. Strontium ranelate: dose-dependent effects in established postmenopausal vertebral osteoporosis--a 2-year randomized placebo controlled trial. *J Clin Endocrinol Metab.* 2002;87(5):2060-2066.

199. Meunier PJ, Roux C, Seeman E, et al. The Effects of Strontium Ranelate on the Risk of Vertebral Fracture in Women with Postmenopausal Osteoporosis. *N Engl J Med.* 2004;350(5):459-468.

200. Beers M, Berkow R, eds. *The Merck Manual of Diagnostic and Therapy: Seventeenth Edition*; 2003.

201. CDC. Prevalence of disability and associated health conditions--United State, 1991-1992. *MMWR.* 1994;43(40):730-739.

202. Jacobs S, Appleton J. *MSM: The Definitive Guide.* Topanga: Freedom Press; 2003.

203. Felson DT, Lawrence RC, Dieppe PA, et al. Osteoarthritis: new insights. Part 1: the disease and its risk factors. *Ann Intern Med.* Oct 17 2000;133(8):635-646.

204. Bland JH, Cooper SM. Osteoarthritis: a review of the cell biology involved and evidence for reversibility. Management rationally related to known genesis and pathophysiology. *Semin Arthritis Rheum.* Nov 1984;14(2):106-133.

205. Helmick C, Lawrence R, Pollard R, Lloyd E, Heyse S. Arthritis and other rheumatic conditions: who is affected now and who will be affected later? *Arthritis Care and Research.* 1995.

206. Lohmander LS. What can we do about osteoarthritis? *Arthritis Res.* 2000;2(2):95 - 100.

207. Silver FH, Bradica G, Tria A. Relationship among biomechanical, biochemical, and cellular changes associated with osteoarthritis. *Crit Rev Biomed Eng.* 2001;29(4):373-391.

208. Smith RL. Degradative enzymes in osteoarthritis. *Front Biosci.* Oct 15 1999;4:D704-712.

209. Sowers M. Epidemiology of risk factors for osteoarthritis: systemic factors. *Curr Opin Rheumatol.* Sep 2001;13(5):447-451.

210. Sinkov V, Cymet T. Osteoarthritis: understanding the pathophysiology, genetics, and treatments. *J Natl Med Assoc.* Jun 2003;95(6):475-482.

211. Rizzo R, Grandolfo M, Godeas C, Jones KW, Vittur F. Calcium, sulfur, and zinc distribution in normal and arthritic articular equine cartilage: a synchrotron radiation-induced X-ray emission (SRIXE) study. *J Exp Zool.* Sep 1 1995;273(1):82-86.

212. Spector TD, Cicuttini F, Baker J, Loughlin J, Hart D. Genetic influences on osteoarthritis in women: a twin study. *BMJ.* April 13, 1996 1996;312(7036):940-943.

213. Lawrence JS, Bremner JM, Bier F. Osteo-arthrosis. Prevalence in the population and relationship between symptoms and x-ray changes. *Ann Rheum Dis.* Jan 1966;25(1):1-24.

214. Baird CL. First-line treatment for osteoarthritis. Part 2: Nonpharmacologic interventions and evaluation. *Orthop Nurs.* Nov-Dec 2001;20(6):13-18; quiz 18-20.

215. Brooks PM, Potter SR, Buchanan WW. NSAID and osteoarthritis--help or hindrance? *J Rheumatol.* Jan-Feb 1982;9(1):3-5.

216. van der Kraan PM, Vitters EL, de Vries BJ, van den Berg WB. High susceptibility of human articular cartilage glycosaminoglycan synthesis to changes in inorganic sulfate availability. *J Orthop Res.* Jul 1990;8(4):565-571.

217. Frankenfield DC, Rowe WA, Cooney RN, Smith JS, Becker D. Limits of body mass index to detect obesity and predict body composition. *Nutrition.* Jan 2001;17(1):26-30.

218. Morris ME, Levy G. Serum concentration and renal excretion by normal adults of inorganic sulfate after acetaminophen, ascorbic acid, or sodium sulfate. *Clin Pharmacol Ther.* Apr 1983;33(4):529-536.

219. Hoffman DA, Wallace SM, Verbeeck RK. Circadian rhythm of serum sulfate levels in man and acetaminophen pharmacokinetics. *Eur J Clin Pharmacol.* 1990;39(2):143-148.

220. Felson DT, Lawrence RC, Hochberg MC, et al. Osteoarthritis: New Insights: Part 2: Treatment Approaches. *Ann Intern Med.* November 7, 2000 2000;133(9):726-737.

221. Ilias I, Vgontzas AN, Provata A, Mastorakos G. Complexity and non-linear description of diurnal cortisol and growth hormone secretory patterns before and after sleep deprivation. *Endocr Regul.* Jun 2002;36(2):63-72.

222. Ferril W. *The Body Heals.* White Fish, MT: Bridge Medical Publishing; 2003.

223. Worthington V. Nutritional quality of organic versus conventional fruits, vegetables and grains. *Journal of Alternative and Complementary Medicine.* 2001;7(2):161-173.

224. Worthington V. Effect of agricultural methods on nutritional quality: a comparison of organic with conventional crops. *Altern Ther Health Med.* Jan 1998;4(1):58-69.

225. Murray M, Pizzorno J. Osteoarthritis. In: Pizzorno J, Murray M, eds. *Textbook of Natural Medicine.* 2d ed: Harcourt Brace and Company; 1999.

226. Gaby A. *Preventing and reversing osteoporosis and arthritis.* Rocklin, CA: Prima Publishing; 1994.

227. Frei B. Reactive oxygen species and antioxidant vitamins: mechanisms of action. *Am J Med.* Sep 26 1994;97(3A):5S-13S; discussion 22S-28S.

228. Darlington LG, Stone TW. Antioxidants and fatty acids in the amelioration of rheumatoid arthritis and related disorders. *Br J Nutr.* Mar 2001;85(3):251-269.

229. Harbige LS. Dietary n-6 and n-3 fatty acids in immunity and autoimmune disease. *Proc Nutr Soc.* Nov 1998;57(4):555-562.

230. Calder PC, Yaqoob P, Thies F, Wallace FA, Miles EA. Fatty acids and lymphocyte functions. *Br J Nutr.* Jan 2002;87 Suppl 1:S31-48.

231. Halpern GM. Anti-inflammatory effects of a stabilized lipid extract of Perna canaliculus (Lyprinol). *Allerg Immunol (Paris).* Sep 2000;32(7):272-278.

232. Deal CL, Schnitzer TJ, Lipstein E, et al. Treatment of arthritis with topical capsaicin: a double-blind trial. *Clin Ther.* May-Jun 1991;13(3):383-395.

233. Singh K. Personal Communication: Clinical Applications of Thymol. Seattle; 2003.

234. Lund-Olesen K, Menander KB. Orgotein: a new anti-inflammatory metalloprotein drug: preliminary evaluation of clinical efficacy and safety in degenerative joint disease. *Curr Ther Res Clin Exp.* Jul 1974;16(7):706-717.

235. Huskisson EC, Scott J. Orgotein in osteoarthritis of the knee joint. *Eur J Rheumatol Inflamm.* 1981;4(2):212-218.

236. Reeves KD, Hassanein K. Randomized prospective double-blind placebo-controlled study of dextrose prolotherapy for knee osteoarthritis with or without ACL laxity. *Altern Ther Health Med.* Mar 2000;6(2):68-74, 77-80.

237. Kimmatkar N, Thawani V, Hingorani L, Khiyani R. Efficacy and tolerability of Boswellia serrata extract in treatment of osteoarthritis of knee--A randomized double blind placebo controlled trial. *Phytomedicine.* 2003;10:3-7.

238. Singh BB, Mishra LC, Vinjamury SP, Aquilina N, Singh VJ, Shepard N. The effectiveness of Commiphora mukul for osteoarthritis of the knee: an outcomes study. *Altern Ther Health Med.* May-Jun 2003;9(3):74-79.

239. Morrison R. *Desktop Guide to Keynotes and Confirmatory Symptoms.* Grass Valley: Hahnemann Clinic Publishing; 1993.

240. Minor MA. Exercise in the treatment of osteoarthritis. *Rheum Dis Clin North Am.* May 1999;25(2):397-415, viii.

241. Garfinkel M, Schumacher HR, Jr. Yoga. *Rheum Dis Clin North Am.* Feb 2000;26(1):125-132, x.

242. Wilens TE, Prince JB, Spencer TJ, Biederman J. Stimulants and Sudden Death: What Is a Physician to Do? *Pediatrics.* 2006;118(3):1215-1219.

243. Wooltorton E. Medications for attention deficit hyperactivity disorder: cardiovascular concerns. *CMAJ.* 2006;175(1):29.

244. Chabas D, Taheri S, Renier C, Mignot E. The Genetics of Narcolepsy. *Annual Review of Genomics and Human Genetics.* 2003;4(1):459-483.

245. Aldrich MS. Diagnostic aspects of narcolepsy. *Neurology.* Feb 1998;50(2 Suppl 1):S2-7.

246. Bassetti C, Aldrich MS. Narcolepsy. *Neurol Clin.* Aug 1996;14(3):545-571.

247. Bassetti C. Narcolepsy. *Curr Treat Options Neurol.* 1999;1(4):291-298.

248. Mignot E. Genetic and familial aspects of narcolepsy. *Neurology.* 1998;50(2 Suppl 1):S16-22.

249. Okun ML, Lin L, Pelin Z, Hong S, Mignot E. Clinical aspects of narcolepsy-cataplexy across ethnic groups. *Sleep.* 2002;25(1):27-35.

250. Overeem S, Mignot E, van Dijk JG, Lammers GJ. Narcolepsy: clinical features, new pathophysiologic insights, and future perspectives. *J Clin Neurophysiol.* 2001;18(2):78-105.

251. Attarian HP. Helping patients who say they cannot sleep. Practical ways to evaluate and treat insomnia. *Postgrad Med.* Mar 2000;107(3):127-142.

252. Lord R, Braley JA, eds. *Laboratory Evaluations for Integrative and Functional Medicine.* 2nd ed. Duluth: Metametrix Institute; 2008.

253. Campistron G, Guiraud R, Cros J, Prat G. Pharmacokinetics of arginine and aspartic acid administered simultaneously in the rat: II. Tissue distribution. *Eur J Drug Metab Pharmacokinet.* 1982;7(4):315-322.

254. Weil-Malherbe H, Krebs HA. Metabolism of amino-acids: The conversion of proline into glutamic acid in kidney. *Biochem J.* Sep 1935;29(9):2077-2081.

255. Kaplan BJ, Simpson JS, Ferre RC, Gorman CP, McMullen DM, Crawford SG. Effective mood stabilization with a chelated mineral supplement: an open-label trial in bipolar disorder. *J Clin Psychiatry.* Dec 2001;62(12):936-944.

256. Montgomery P, Richardson AJ. Omega-3 fatty acids for bipolar disorder. *Cochrane Database Syst Rev.* 2008(2):CD005169.

257. Lakhan SE, Vieira KF. Nutritional therapies for mental disorders. *Nutr J.* 2008;7:2.

258. Lord R, Bralley J. Chapter 6: Organic Acids. In: Lord R, Bralley J, eds. *Laboratory Evaluations for Integrative and Functional Medicine*. Duluth: Metametrix Institute; 2008:319-412.

259. Mansfield LE, Vaughan TR, Waller SF, Haverly RW, Ting S. Food allergy and adult migraine: double-blind and mediator confirmation of an allergic etiology. *Ann Allergy*. Aug 1985;55(2):126-129.

260. Carter CM, Egger J, Soothill JF. A dietary management of severe childhood migraine. *Hum Nutr Appl Nutr*. Aug 1985;39(4):294-303.

261. Hughes EC, Gott PS, Weinstein RC, Binggeli R. Migraine: a diagnostic test for etiology of food sensitivity by a nutritionally supported fast and confirmed by long-term report. *Ann Allergy*. Jul 1985;55(1):28-32.

262. Monro J, Brostoff J, Carini C, Zilkha K. Food allergy in migraine. Study of dietary exclusion and RAST. *Lancet*. Jul 5 1980;2(8184):1-4.

263. Grant EC. Food allergies and migraine. *Lancet*. May 5 1979;1(8123):966-969.

264. Thomas J, Tomb E, Thomas E, Faure G. Migraine treatment by oral magnesium intake and correction of the irritation of buccofacial and cervical muscles as a side effect of mandibular imbalance. *Magnes Res*. Jun 1994;7(2):123-127.

265. Facchinetti F, Sances G, Borella P, Genazzani AR, Nappi G. Magnesium prophylaxis of menstrual migraine: effects on intracellular magnesium. *Headache*. May 1991;31(5):298-301.

266. Schoenen J, Lenaerts M, Bastings E. High-dose riboflavin as a prophylactic treatment of migraine: results of an open pilot study. *Cephalalgia*. Oct 1994;14(5):328-329.

267. Neustadt J, Pieczenik SR. Medication-induced mitochondrial damage and disease. *Mol Nutr Food Res*. Jul 2008;52(7):780-788.

268. Aw TY, Jones DP. Nutrient supply and mitochondrial function. *Annu Rev Nutr*. 1989;9:229-251.

269. Atamna H, Liu J, Ames BN. Heme Deficiency Selectively Interrupts Assembly of Mitochondrial Complex IV in Human Fibroblasts. Relevance to aging. *J. Biol. Chem*. 2001;276(51):48410-48416.

270. Saper RB, Kales SN, Paquin J, et al. Heavy Metal Content of Ayurvedic Herbal Medicine Products. *JAMA*. 2004;292(23):2868-2873.

271. Shrestha M, Greenberg MI. Lead poisoning derived from Ayurvedic medication. (Abstract). *(Abstract).* 2002;40(5):678(671).

272. Caraccio TR, McGuigan M, Mofenson HC. Chronic arsenic (As) toxicity from Chitosan[R] supplement.(Abstract). *(Abstract).* 2002;40(5):644(641).

273. Ernst E, Thompson Coon J. Heavy metals in traditional Chinese medicines: a systematic review. *Clin Pharmacol Ther.* 2001;70(6):552-560.

274. Gurib-Fakim A. Medicinal plants: traditions of yesterday and drugs of tomorrow. *Mol Aspects Med.* Feb 2006;27(1):1-93.

275. Liu YK, Tipton CM, Matthes RD, Bedford TG, Maynard JA, Walmer HC. An in situ study of the influence of a sclerosing solution in rabbit medial collateral ligaments and its junction strength. *Connect Tissue Res.* 1983;11(2-3):95-102.

276. Ongley MJ, Klein RG, Dorman TA, Eek BC, Hubert LJ. A new approach to the treatment of chronic low back pain. *Lancet.* Jul 18 1987;2(8551):143-146.

277. Alternative treatments. Dealing with chronic pain. *Mayo Clin Health Lett.* Apr 2005;23(4):1-3.

Index

Page numbers marked with an "f" indicate figures; those with a "t" indicate tables.

R